Creating with God

Grace and Peace,
Sarah Jobe

Sarah Jobe

Creating with God

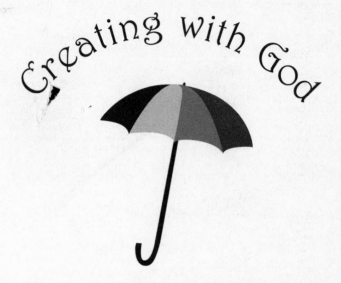

THE HOLY CONFUSING

BLESSEDNESS OF PREGNANCY

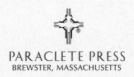

PARACLETE PRESS
BREWSTER, MASSACHUSETTS

Creating with God: The Holy Confusing Blessedness of Pregnancy

Copyright © 2011 by Sarah Jobe

ISBN 978-1-55725-922-6

Library of Congress Cataloging-in-Publication Data

Jobe, Sarah, 1981-
  Creating with God : the holy confusing blessedness of pregnancy / Sarah Jobe.
    p. cm.
  Includes bibliographical references (p.   ).
  ISBN 978-1-55725-922-6 (paper back)
  1. Jobe, Sarah, 1981–2. Pregnant women—Religious life. 3. Pregnancy—Religious aspects—Christianity. I. Title.
  BV4529.18.J53 2011
  248.8′431—dc23   2011017343

10 9 8 7 6 5 4 3 2 1

Published by Paraclete Press
Brewster, Massachusetts
www.paracletepress.com
Printed in the United States of America

To Naomi and Fay,

who held my fingers in their sticky hands
as we all grew up together.
I realized my own worth as I marveled at yours.

And to Dan,

who has scooted ever closer to the edge of the bed
to make room for us all.
I see Jesus in you.

CONTENTS

PART THREE

Birthing the Fruit of the Spirit

Author's Note

AS I WAS FINISHING THIS BOOK, my best friend Holly was carefully boxing up her maternity clothes. Holly explained to me that she actually cried while putting them in the attic, realizing that she didn't get to be pregnant any more. Holly can't wait for baby number three and the opportunity to take her maternity clothes out of storage.

I love Holly. But I think you should know, right from the start, that I'm not that type of pregnant woman. After back-to-back pregnancies, I gave away every stitch of maternity clothing I owned in the hopes that any future children might think twice before nestling into the wall of my uterus. I won't say that I hated pregnancy. But I can't say that I loved it either. Pregnancy was the most difficult endeavor I have ever undertaken.

Don't misunderstand; nothing actually went wrong during my pregnancies. According to my midwives, my pregnancies were "uncomplicated." But I have decided that *uncomplicated* is one of those words that just doesn't apply to even the most straightforward of births. Pregnancy is the most complicated mess I've ever gotten myself into.

I don't know what I expected from pregnancy. I had heard that pregnancy was a blessing, and I think I hoped to feel special, encouraged, or invigorated by being blessed. Instead, I felt exhausted. As in, someone peel me off the floor and have the decency to deposit me in my bed exhausted. I think I hoped for some sort of warm maternal feeling to well up within me. But the only thing welling up on a regular basis was heartburn. I had hoped to meet physical challenges with grace. Instead, I found myself collapsing daily onto my bathroom floor, the neighbors' couch, or the sidewalk in front of my office. I was a mess of tears, snot, backache, and self-doubt. Not exactly graceful.

Perhaps the hardest thing about pregnancy was that I couldn't figure out where God was in all of it. I was in the midst of the most transformative event of my life and God seemed nowhere to be found. I was too tired for my traditional spiritual disciplines. Worship services seemed designed for nonpregnant people who could sit in a pew without painfully swollen ankles and raging sciatic nerve pain. And any part of Christianity that had to do with being an energetic and cheerful giver seemed about as possible as fitting into my pre-pregnancy jeans.

This book was born from my attempt to cling to the idea that pregnancy is a blessing in spite of my experience to the contrary. I began the book wondering how God could be present in pregnancy *in spite of* back pain, financial stress, hormonal shifts, and constipation. But as I wrote, I have learned a startling truth. God is not present in pregnancy *in spite of* all the crap (and I mean that in the most literal sense). God is present in pregnancy at precisely the places that seem least divine.

This book is an attempt to name how pregnant women are co-creators with God at precisely the moment in which we are pooping on the delivery table. I will claim that pregnant women are the image of Jesus among us not in spite of varicose veins but because of them. I will explore how the practices we take up on behalf of our growing babies train us in the very practices we need to live a life of faith.

Pregnancy is at the heart of God's work in the world. Pregnant women are the image of God among us. But those truths are sometimes hard to see. This book is an attempt to wipe off the mirrors we use to see ourselves. I hope you will go from this book able to see yourself differently. I hope you might learn to see God when you look in the mirror.

There is no need to read the chapters of this book in the order given. When I was pregnant, I experienced an odd upheaval in my reading style. One day I would wake up completely obsessed with birth positions and know that I could not possibly eat breakfast until I had scoured our birth books for a list of all the possible positions in which I might labor. A few days of intense research would ensue (with attendant birth ball purchase), and then the interest would be gone. A few days later I might wake up needing to know everything about fetal hiccups.

Follow your interests when deciding which chapters to read. The chapters are arranged theologically and have a certain sense. The first section describes the ways that women partner with God in the work of pregnancy. The second section describes specific ways that pregnant women become the image of Christ among us. The last section describes how the practices of pregnancy might train us in the spiritual disciplines we need for a life of faith.

But pregnant brains don't always need theological sense. Sometimes we just want to know about ultrasounds, and on that day you should read chapter 3.

You might also want a warning that chapters 4, 6, and 8 contain stories of loss and difficulty in childbirth. There were many days during my pregnancies where the last thing I needed was even the first hint of a sad story. Avoid chapters 4, 6, and 8 on those days.

Whatever order you choose, I pray that these chapters might be a gift, ideally a more straightforward sort of gift than pregnancy itself. I still can't bring myself to say that I love pregnancy. But deep down, I really do. Pregnancy is a place where heaven and earth meet and constipation takes on cosmic significance. What's not to love?

PART ONE
Mothering with God the Father

1
Co-Creating with God

—

"I have created a man with God!"

GENESIS 4:1

I ATTENDED MY FIVE-YEAR COLLEGE REUNION four months pregnant, with my one-year-old daughter in tow. I knew that none of my immediate friends had children. I knew that most of my classmates were in the first, fast-paced years of careers they had been anticipating for a lifetime. I knew that I had not lost the weight of my first pregnancy before getting pregnant with my second and that I was in that awkward period where I didn't really look pregnant per se, more like severely bloated, or maybe like someone who had been dipping a bit too generously into the postdinner ice cream carton.

I thought I had taken these facts into account when planning for the reunion. While I could still fit into some pre-pregnancy clothes, I planned to wear only my trendiest maternity outfits—the ones with empire waists and expanding ties in the back. I figured I would give my nonpregnant peers every indication that I was pregnant and not just an extremely liberal ice cream eater (or rather, that I was pregnant, and *thus understandably* an extremely liberal ice cream eater).

I had thought about the most impressive ways of narrating my ten-hour-a-week job. I had reminded myself that other people didn't want to hear about how my daughter Naomi had started walking on the early side and was in the 97th percentile for her height (a clear sign of an ingenious, generally spectacular person, if you ask me). I had committed to be the energetic, charismatic woman I hoped people remembered from college . . . only pregnant and toting a baby.

I had no idea what I was in for.

We got into town and drove immediately to a reception for an academic program that had been a huge part of my college experience. My closest friends had been in the program, and I figured it would be the safest place to experiment with being the only pregnant mom in a room. Within the first hour, I heard about a woman's career on Wall Street, one man's backpacking trip throughout Europe, and another man's success in preventing communicable diseases in a country I wasn't sure I had ever heard of before.

My complete mental breakdown came as I was listening to a perfectly coiffed woman named Alyssa explain that she had recently become a "personal life assistant." My husband,

Dan, had clearly forgotten his instructions to usher me out of conversations like this one. Alyssa explained that she had just taken the red-eye from San Francisco, and I wondered how one could sit on a plane overnight and emerge without a single wrinkle on a silk skirt designed by someone with a well-known Italian name in a size that I couldn't wear even before back-to-back pregnancies.

"Now what, exactly, is a life assistant?" I asked. I should have seen the silk skirt, made the obvious assumptions, and found a way to exit the conversation. But I honestly had no idea what a life assistant was, and if it happened to be some sort of social service, I was quite sure I could use one. With one baby and another on the way, I needed all the assistance I could get.

Alyssa's eyes sparkled as she launched into an explanation about people with lots of money but very little time maximizing their social potential. I was really only half listening to Alyssa because the other half of me was listening to the garbled beginnings of speech bubbling up from the one-year-old attached to my leg. Even with the distraction, it quickly became clear that folks like me, those with both little time *and* little money, did not have the privilege of life assistants.

I could see Dan sampling the free cheeses across the room, oblivious to my impending breakdown. Naomi's half-speech was becoming more intense, and I looked down just in time to see her finish smearing her bit of free cheese across my only pair of black maternity capris. Just when the comparison between Alyssa's silk skirt and my cheesy capris was becoming completely unbearable, my best friend swept into the room. She yelled my name and ran through the crowd, pushing the silk skirt away with a needed hug. I pretended that my tears were from joy at seeing her again. As we headed to our favorite ice cream shop, I couldn't help but think, "What am I doing with my life?"

Pregnancy is a blessing. At least, that's what people told pregnant women throughout my life. I heard it when I got pregnant with my first child. Of course, when I got pregnant *again* eight months after the birth of my first child, the "blessing" line morphed into something more like, "You've got your work cut out for you. But of course, children are such a blessing."

The rhetoric at my reunion was no different. I spent the weekend hearing a continual round of, "Congratulations!" I also heard a heavy dose of, "You are so lucky!" coupled with covetous looks and not-so-hidden jabs delivered to the ribs of husbands and boyfriends who seemed eager to excuse themselves to the bar, where, of course, there were no obnoxious pregnant ladies giving their partners "ideas." I even heard the occasional, "You look happier than you've ever looked!" Which made me seriously worry about what sort of impression I made in college. But as my ankles swelled up in Virginia's June heat and I missed the reunion nightlife due to sheer exhaustion (and Naomi's bed time), I couldn't help but think, "Remind me again exactly how pregnancy is a blessing?"

Everyone seemed to embrace the party line that pregnancy is something to be celebrated. But I noticed that of the hundreds of women there, only one other woman was pregnant. Somehow, the blessing of pregnancy wasn't yet enough to lure others away from careers and travel and social engagements that are much more difficult to do with a baby either in utero or out.

And from my position as the lone pregnant woman, it seemed that perhaps my peers had made the better decision. Pregnancy is hard work, but it affords none of the possibility for advancement that careers offer. The work of pregnancy is not paid. There are no awards or systems for external recognition. It's not something to write on one's resume. Pregnancy is something of a relationship, but it's not like investing in the mutuality of friendships or romantic relationships. I felt like I was giving a lot more than I was getting from my relationships with my unborn children. Pregnancy requires an entire life change, much of which is about giving up basic enjoyments like wine, cheese, Advil, and the possibility of walking short distances free of sciatic nerve pain.

We insist that pregnancy is a blessing, but women are waiting longer and longer to get pregnant. And it's no wonder. Women have more and more to lose, and neither society nor the church have taken time to name the specific ways that pregnancy is work worth undertaking.

Eve is the first woman to ever give birth. She delivers a little boy named Cain, and she exclaims, "I have created a man with God!" Even if you know that these words come from Genesis 4:1, you won't find them in most English Bibles. The King James Version has Eve exclaim, "I have gotten a man from the Lord," as if God sent Cain in a brightly wrapped package complete with bow and operating instructions. In the New International Version, Eve says, "With the help of the Lord I have brought forth a man." Some translations like the Revised Standard Version combine the two, saying, "I have gotten a man with the help of the LORD." Across the board, English translators seem to avoid the straightforward meaning of these four Hebrew words: I have created a man with God.

The verb that Eve uses to describe what she has done is not the standard word used for labor and delivery. Eve uses the word *create* to describe her work. And Eve says nothing of having God's "help" in the matter. She uses a short preposition that very plainly means "with." She doesn't create with God's help. She creates *with* God. In her joy at giving birth, Eve boldly claims her status as a co-creator. Her claim is startling.

Her claim is even more startling if you've read the three chapters leading up to her exclamation. The first thing the Bible says about God is that God is Creator. Chapters 1–3 of Genesis take time to outline the details of God's creative activity. This Israelite creation narrative would have stood alongside other creation narratives of the time, boldly claiming that the God of Israel, and no others gods, created the heaven, earth, sun, moon, and stars. Only the God of Israel can claim creative powers. And then comes Eve. She is one of God's creations, and yet she claims that she too has the power to create alongside God.

Even more startling is that she claims this creative power at the moment of childbearing. Just a few verses prior, the pains of childbearing had been named as curse. Genesis 2–3 tells the story of how Adam and Eve disobeyed God's command and ate the fruit of the tree of knowledge of good and evil. When God finds out about the trespass, the curses start flying. The serpent who tempted them is cursed. The ground is cursed. Death is introduced to human life, and Adam and Eve are sent out of the garden. Pain is introduced into childbearing. Genesis 3:16 says, "I will make your pains in childbearing very severe; with painful labor you will give birth to children."

The story of Eve's labor and delivery is the very next story in the Bible. If I were writing it, I would highlight the pain that Eve experienced. I would make extra effort to show how the curse was fulfilled in this first experience of labor. I might even throw in a little video footage, so everyone would be sure to hear Eve's groans. Ideally, Eve would give a rousing speech of repentance as she holds little Cain in her arms.

But the Bible says no such thing. Not a word is given about birth pains, even though elsewhere the Bible is quick to associate labor with pain. Instead of pain, the writers of Scripture pass down Eve's strong, joyful exclamation, "I have created a man with God!"

Eve knows something that we are slow to admit. Eve realizes, as she experiences the power of pregnancy and labor, that she is involved in God's work. Eve knows God as the creator of heaven and earth. Eve knows God as the one who created her and her partner Adam. And then she finds herself creating a whole new human being, too. She can't help but notice that this is the sort of work her God is busy with. And as she brings that new life into the world, she is filled with pride at having taken on divine activity. She has been God's hands and feet and womb in the world. She has been given the gift of doing God's work, and the knowledge of it changes her curse to blessing.

Eve names her son "Cain." The word in Hebrew sounds like the word Eve used earlier for "create." Cain's name will forever tell her story. His name will testify to her power as a creator. His name will remind him that his birth was not a curse but a blessing because it gave his mother the opportunity to partner with God. The truth is, each of us could name our newborn "Cain."

My family will not let me forget that I used to want to name my child Chlorene. When I was twelve years old, I announced this choice to my family. Before announcing it, I hadn't given a thought to the fact that "Chlorene" sounds exactly like "chlorine." I thought the vowel sounds in the word rolled together beautifully. I loved the way my mouth felt saying it. Of course, the announcement was met with a brief silence before my younger siblings broke into uproarious laughter that has continued to this day whenever the subject of baby names is brought up.

After a few months of daily ridicule, I rescinded my choice of name. Chlorene might sound lovely, but I couldn't name my child after a pool-cleansing chemical. The meaning of a name matters.

Pregnant women spend hours researching baby names. From name books to online lists, from family histories to the Bible, anything is a potential source for that perfect name. Dan and I searched for a name that would give our child a vision for her life. We wanted a name with a story. We wanted an inspirational name. We wanted a name that would connect our child to her family and to the God that we knew loved her even more than we did.

We named our first child Naomi Ruth. We liked the idea of a biblical name, but we didn't want our daughter to feel locked into one biblical character. By choosing two characters from the same story, we hoped to offer the story instead of the characters as inspiration for our daughter's life. The book of Ruth is a story of intergenerational friendship between women. We prayed that Naomi would be gifted with such friendship in her life. The story is about extended family crossing cultural divides to sustain one another. We prayed Naomi would have the courage to reach across some of those same social divisions.

We named our second daughter Fay Marie. Fay is my grandmother's name. Fay also sounds like the Spanish word for "faith." Faith is my mother-in-law's maiden name. We hoped that Fay might one day find the faith in God that has nourished our lives and our marriage. We prayed that she would remain connected to both sides of her family. Marie is a common middle name among my husband's very Catholic relatives. Marie reminds of mother Mary. We prayed that Fay would find a way to embrace both her Baptist and Catholic heritage. We prayed that she would find strong women like Mary to guide her through her life.

We gave both of our daughters the last name Schwankl-Jobe. We don't pretend that it sounds good. It sounds something like a Polish sausage gone wrong. We have learned that you have to be at least three years old to even begin pronouncing it. We hope our daughters will be able to bear the jokes they will no doubt receive in middle school over this name. But we wanted our daughters to carry the histories of both of our families within them. We wanted them to be reminded, every time they introduced themselves, from whence they came.

Names matter. The words we use to name people and things convey meaning. It matters if we say that Eve "acquired" a child "with the help" of God. That is different than saying that Eve and God are co-creators.

This book is about naming. But it's not about naming our babies. It's more about naming ourselves. In this book, I will muster up the courage of Eve, the courage that motherhood has given me, to make some bold and joyous proclamations. I will name the work of pregnancy as the work of God. I will name the pregnant women around me as the image of Christ. I will call the pains of pregnancy "spiritual disciplines."

My prayer is that as we hear ourselves named something new, we will see our phenomenal worth and be encouraged. Naming pregnancy as the work of God has the power to change the curses of it into blessing.

I wish I had known that at the college reunion. I realized over the ensuing year that I didn't know how to answer the question, "So, what are you doing these days?" Because pregnancy doesn't fit on a resume, I had excluded it as a valid answer. Instead, I would answer sort of sheepishly, "Well, I work about ten hours a week, and then, you know, I spend a good bit of time with these little ones," gesturing to the children that were no doubt clinging to various parts of my body. I would then feel pathetic and self-conscious as my conversation partners explained all that they were accomplishing in their fifty-hour-a-week jobs.

But now I'm learning to embrace Eve's bold claim. What I have actually been doing is creating people with God. Now my answer to what I do goes something like, "Well, in my spare time I work for a nonprofit, but I have focused most of my energy on creating two new human beings. It's exhausting work. But I love it." Okay, so I don't always say it out loud. I haven't quite embraced the fullness of Eve's audacious sass. But I at least remind myself of it in the space where I used to feel pathetic and unaccomplished. And it has made all the difference.

2
Delighting in the Details

"You are precious and honored in my sight,
and . . . I love you."

ISAIAH 43:4

MY HUSBAND TOOK OFF WORK the day of our ultrasound. We drove twenty-five minutes together to a hospital in Chapel Hill. There were closer hospitals, but this one partnered with the free-standing midwifery practice we had chosen for the birth of our first daughter. We rode in excited silence, smiling at each other across the stick shift of my husband's car. I turned on the radio and began changing the stations impatiently. No song seemed fit for the prelude to our first glimpse of our first child. I cut it off again.

"Do you think she'll be a girl?" I asked. The question was actually more of a squeal than a question. I could barely contain my unabashed hope.

"We will be blessed to have a boy or a girl," answered my politically correct, frustratingly calm husband.

This exchange had become something of a mantra between us in the past months. While I knew it was unmotherly and horribly biased, I longed for a girl the way I longed for my mother's cinnamon rolls on Christmas morning. I still don't believe that Dan had no opinion on the subject, but he never deviated from the parental party line that a child of either gender would be delightful.

We settled back into silence. The quiet in the car seemed oddly wrapped around the din of thoughts drumming through my head. "Will the baby be healthy? Will she be moving? Will we be able to see what she looks like? How big will she be? She's not a she! Not a she! Not a she! I will be happy with a boy. I will be happy with a boy. A tiny, lovely, fun, roly-poly boy . . . What will I do with a boy?"

I looked down and realized I was pumping my legs back and forth, a nervous habit I picked up from my mother. The motion is the same as the one you do on those exercise machines meant to work your inner thighs. Except I pump my legs much faster than one can achieve on the exercise machine, neurotically fast, as if am trying to pump out the barrage of questions clogging up my brain. My leg pump seemed to be broken because the questions weren't going anywhere.

"Will she look like me?" My question broke the silence.

Unphased by my excitement, Dan replied, "*He* or she will be lucky to look like you."

I rolled my eyes, but didn't completely overlook the compliment. "He must have just read the chapter on how to be a calm and effective partner to a neurotic pregnant woman on the way to an ultrasound," I thought.

Both of us had been pouring over the veritable library of birthing books littering our bedroom floor. We wanted to know what to do, how to eat, what to buy, and how to be prepared. But in truth, all of that was not what kept me turning the pages night after night. In those early months, I read for one reason only. I wanted to know my baby.

I was desperate for any news, and while the authors of those books hadn't met my baby any more than I had, they certainly seemed to know a lot about what *he or she* was doing. They knew what size she was each week. They informed me when she had grown from the size of a pea to the size of a kidney bean. They told me when his little hands grew finger buds, and when his little lungs began to work. They told me when he or she had become a he or she, when her eyelids formed, and when he began to practice sucking. Those books seemed to know details about my baby that I hungered to know, and I delighted in every detail they delivered.

If a picture is worth a thousand words, an ultrasound is worth ten thousand baby books. While I had delighted to learn of my baby's finger buds, now I had the chance to see my particular baby's fingers. I wondered if they would be long and elegant like my husband's grandmother, or short and stubby like mine. Maybe they would be a completely new fusion of the two. I couldn't wait to see them.

After the usual round of paperwork and waiting rooms, we were directed to a dimly lit room. I was invited to recline on something like a dentist's chair, and I remember being annoyed by the way the attendant folded up the bottom of my shirt and unceremoniously squirted a blob of gel on my stomach. My midwives had always squirted the gel onto the handheld device. Somehow that seemed less invasive than a direct squirt on my stomach. I was lost in my own analysis of why the blob of gel was bothering me so much when my husband gasped. I looked up to a blurry black and white image. The screen pulsed and skipped with life. One pattern flashed after another.

"This one's a mover!" exclaimed the attendant. The baby kicked and flipped, and the attendant took a few minutes to orient herself to the movement. My husband squeezed my hand. His face broke into a huge grin and tears flowed down his cheeks. I couldn't take my eyes off the screen to smile back, so I squeezed his hand in mine.

The attendant began cataloguing and measuring the baby's parts. She would freeze the screen every so often and type a word across the image. Kidney . . . Heart . . . Brain . . . We watched the parade of our child's parts with an awe that no Macy's Thanksgiving Day extravaganza has ever evoked. The attendant froze the screen again and began to type, "I-M-A-G-I-R" My husband began to cheer and looked at me as if I should be more excited about this image than the last.

"What?" I asked.

"Read the screen!" he laughed.

"Imagirl?" I asked.

"I'm a girl!" he corrected, launching into an unnecessarily detailed account about how I really wanted a girl and couldn't imagine having a boy, as if the ultrasound technician really needed to know how far I had strayed from unbiased parental love for all children. But I could barely feel my annoyance underneath the fleecy blanket of joy that had begun to settle over my body. Her little girl parts were flanked by thighs that looked just like my own. They were the "Chilton thighs" that my mother and aunts complained would always be big no matter how skinny the rest of their bodies were. My daughter had my thighs.

The technician warned that a frontal view of her face might be scary, looking more like a skeleton than a person. But the image that appeared revealed a little face with my husband's jaw line. The fleecy blanket of joy settled on us with a palpable weight, covering me and the little girl who we explored and admired. In the profile picture, I found that she had my nose, a round ball of a nose that is markedly different from the angular slope of my husband's.

Through the entire ultrasound the baby kicked and squirmed, turning entirely over at one point. She covered her ears and pounded her fist in the air. The technician captured one image of our daughter holding her triumphant little fist over her head.

"She looks like a punk rocker," beamed my husband.

"No, she's demanding power for the people," I corrected. We smiled together, cherishing this little daughter who already had so much spunk and zeal for life.

When I was in college, my grandmother gave me a framed quotation to hang on my wall. It read, "I have called you by name, Sarah. You are mine. You are precious and honored in my sight, and I love you." The phrases are taken from Isaiah 43. As I struggled with body image, self-doubt, and all the usual identity crises of young women in their early twenties, I would gaze at that quotation on my wall. I would read it over and over again, repeating it to myself when my worries kept me awake at night. I could barely believe that God thought so highly of me, yet I clung to that truth as if it were a neon orange life preserver.

The quotation suggests that each of us is special in God's sight. God knows and remembers my particular name, out of all the names of God's children. God knows me as an individual. God loves me, not in some vague way, but for the quirkiness of who I am. I had trouble understanding this kind of love because I didn't love my own voice and thighs and pride and intellect as much as God seemed to. But I also had trouble understanding this kind of love because I had never given this kind of love to another person.

Pregnancy taught me how to delight in the details of another human being. Marriage had given me a window into this sort of delight, but motherhood settled me into this kind of loving as a way of life. Even before I could see or hear my child, I found her details delightful. I delighted to experience the parts of her that seemed like most other babies. I delighted to learn what made her special. I was intrigued when her hiccups created rhythmic surges in my tummy. I experimented with what might cause those tremors with the curiosity of a scientist measuring seismic waves.

Near the end of my first pregnancy, I swore up and down that my daughter was twirling her hands at the opening of my cervix. The twirling motion was unmistakable and odd. It made me laugh and gave me goose bumps. Everyone around me scoffed, sure that at ten days past my due date my imagination was creating a mental image of my daughter unsuccessfully trying to claw her way out. But to my delight, my daughter was born with her hands tucked underneath her chin. Within minutes of birth and for months after, she would twirl her hands in just the circles I had felt. She even kept the habit of twirling them right up beside her face.

I find this detail about my daughter completely endearing. The way she twirls her hands is not a virtue. I cannot brag about it as a sign of intellect or creativity or compassion. Her hand twirling does not take skill. She doesn't even seem aware of this detail about herself. And yet it is precious in my sight. It is a detail that I cherish and hold in my heart. It is a bit of knowledge about my daughter that I feel lucky to know and have experienced.

Because I love my daughter this way, I can begin to understand the way that God loves me. God loves the details that make me who I am. God adores even the details that are not virtues, or strengths, or good qualities. God loves the mundane things about us. God loves our quirks. God loves the way we hold our heads when we are confused about something, the way we shrug our shoulders when we are excited, and the expressions on our faces when we are deep in thought. "You are precious and honored in my sight, and I love you." God whispers the words as a mother whispers to her child.

We get a glimpse of the way God delights in the details of creation in the book of Job. We know the story of Job for its question of why bad things happen to good people. Job is a faithful servant of God. In a bet with Satan, God allows Job to lose his wealth, his health, and even his children. Job's friends are convinced that Job has done something to deserve this suffering. Job's wife encourages him to curse God and die. Job insists on his own innocence and demands an explanation from God.

God hears Job and responds, but God's response is not an explanation. Instead, God launches into a monologue about God's creatures. The speech has nothing to do with Job. For four chapters, God goes on ad nauseam about the delightful details found in creation, even self-describing as a mother, "from whose womb comes the ice . . . who gives birth to the frost from the heavens?" (38:29). God describes oxen and lions and ravens. God describes each creature in turn, noting what makes each creature unique with the care and attention of one who has gazed at those creatures with a mother's untiring eyes. God shares the following description with Job, saying:

> The wings of the ostrich flap joyfully,
> though they cannot compare with the wings
>> and feathers of the stork.
> She lays her eggs on the ground
> and lets them warm in the sand,
> unmindful that a foot may crush them,
> that some wild animal may trample them.
> She treats her young harshly, as if they were not hers;
> She cares not that her labor was in vain,
> for God did not endow her with wisdom
> or give her a share of good sense.
> Yet when she spreads her feathers to run,
> she laughs at horse and rider.
> Do you give the horse his strength
> or clothe his neck with a flowing mane?
> Do you make him leap like a locust,

striking terror with his proud snorting?
It paws fiercely, rejoicing in his strength,
and charges into the fray.
He laughs at fear, afraid of nothing;
he does not shy away from the sword. (39:13–22)

God goes on and on like this. God describes the specifics of each creature with a loving attention to detail. The details of the description reveal that God does indeed know and call each animal by name. God even describes what might be considered negative attributes about the way the ostrich treats her young, but then paints a glorious image of that same ostrich speeding over the earth.

When reading Job there is a temptation to skip these passages. They seem beside the point. We want to know what God has to say about Job's suffering, and God insists on blathering on like a mother in love with her newborn child. We want answers. God wants us to glimpse the way we are loved.

I take time to listen to God's description in Job because I know what it means to be the one describing the details of my child until the eyes of my listener glaze over. I recognize God's mind-numbingly detailed account as the way I describe my children. Job asks God a deep theological question. God answers, "Have you seen the latest picture of my babies?" I am both proud and embarrassed to admit that in the past years of pregnancy and child rearing I have answered people the way God answers Job.

Perhaps the revelation of God's giddy and extravagant love for the ostrich is the best answer Job could receive. In Matthew's Gospel, Jesus tells his disciples, "Are not two sparrows sold for a penny? Yet not one of them will fall to the ground outside your Father's care. And even the very hairs of your head are all numbered. So don't be afraid; you are worth more than many sparrows" (10:29–31).

The God who adores the ostrich knows every hair on Job's head. The adoration God expresses for the ostrich cannot compare to the way God knows and loves Job. God invites Job to witness the way God delights in the beautiful absurdity of each creature. Behind God's description of love for the ostrich God whispers to Job, "I have called you by name. You are mine. You are precious and honored in my sight, and I love you."

These words of adoration appear in a very complex passage in the book of Isaiah. God's people have rejected God and chosen to worship the work of their own hands. God has punished them by allowing Babylon to conquer their homeland entirely. The people of Israel were led out from their homes in chains to live as exiles in Babylon. In this passage, God rails angrily about his children's betrayal. In the next breath, God lovingly calls his children back home. We try to avoid the angry, judgmental God that we find in the Bible, opting for passages about God's radical love and grace. But in Isaiah, God's seething anger and deep adoration cannot be untangled. We have to make sense of them together. Isaiah does it by imagining God as a mom.

I lay on my back, my mind and body numb from shock. Both of my hands rested on the warm, squishy lump that the midwife had deposited on my chest. I couldn't see her, but she felt like a wet puppy—one of those wrinkled puppies with rolls of extra skin. I remembered the woman in the birth video I had watched weeks before. She had delivered an eloquent speech to her newborn son, exclaiming, "My son! My little son! Welcome to the world! I am so glad you are here!" It had seemed like a good way to welcome someone into the world, and I had resolved to welcome my daughter with a similar speech. But now my legs shook with fatigue, and my tongue was thick with exhaustion.

"I should say something," I thought to myself. But my mind seemed to have had the breath knocked out of it. I couldn't make sense of the pain radiating through my hips and the wet puppy-lump resting on my chest.

"I brought you into this world, and I can take you out of it." I had heard the phrase before, said sternly at unruly children, said with raised eyebrows as a warning, said mockingly with a smile. I had heard it, but I had never understood it. It seemed such a harsh thing to say to a child. How could giving birth entitle a woman to that kind of sway over her child's life? As I lay on my back, reeling from the experience of labor, the phrase floated into my head. "I brought you into this world," I thought. I might not be able to justify the second half of the saying, but all of a sudden I could imagine myself using it.

Isaiah imagines God as just this sort of mother. God is the one who "creates and forms" God's people. God is the "Redeemer, who formed you in the womb" (44:24). God has brought her children to life, and she delights in the details of their existence. But her children have not returned the favor. While God has called her children by name, they have not called upon her. While she has labored to give them birth, they have not wearied themselves for her. They have instead wearied her with their offenses (43:22–24). While she has provided them food and everything needed for life, they have refused to bring her offerings. While she has called them "precious and honored in my sight," they have refused to "[honor] me with your sacrifices" (43:4, 23).

While God delights in her people the way a mother delights in her children, Isaiah reveals that God wants to be loved the same way in return. God desires that we would turn our delight back around on her. When we don't, God gets mad.

We often imagine this angry God as a king or despot, as a disciplinarian or father. But Isaiah knows that this angry

God is a mother. God rails at the unruly children she labored to birth. She barks at them with the ferocity of her love, "I brought you into this world, and I can take you out of it!" And in the next breath she cries out, "Bring my sons from afar and my daughters from the ends of the earth—everyone who is called by my name, whom I created for my glory, whom I formed and made" (43:6–7). When we understand God as mother, we understand how God's anger at betrayal can never be separated from God's deep delight in the children she has labored to bring forth.

This passage in Isaiah ends with God taking time to delight specifically in her child Cyrus. Cyrus is a king whom God plans to use to bring Israel back to their homeland. This plan seems straightforward enough, but scholars have worried and worried over God's choice of Cyrus because Cyrus is not a Jew. Cyrus does not acknowledge God, and yet God "calls him by name" just as God calls Israel. God seems to delight in Cyrus, just as God delights in Israel. While scholars have difficulty understanding why God would delight in and choose a pagan king, Isaiah knows that God's love is like the ever-expanding love of a mother. Delight in one child doesn't diminish the awe of learning the details of a second, third, or fourth little one.

As we drove to the ultrasound of our second child, only a year after the birth of our first, the questions crowding my brain were different. My leg pumping was just as ferocious.

I still longed for a girl, and I was even more embarrassed by my longing. Surely, after having one girl, I could be satisfied with a boy! But I had visions of matching dresses, a shared room, and a pair of best friends who would enter womanhood together.

"Will she look like Naomi?" I asked.

"*He* or she will be beautiful in *his* or her own way," answered my husband. He was still toeing the parental party line.

This time I was prepared for the blob of gel. I had my eyes fixed on the screen before the technician could even find our child. The black and white image appeared. It pulsed lightly, but there was no skipping on the screen. Our baby rested as calmly as her father does. When the technician showed us her profile, I gasped.

"She looks so different from Naomi!" I exclaimed.

"How can you tell?" asked Dan.

"Look at her nose!" I pointed to the angular slope that marks Dan's family. "Naomi's nose was nothing like that."

We learned that we would have a second daughter, and this time my eyes filled with tears. The technician captured an image of the underside of her foot. I memorized that image, and to my delight, Fay entered the world with the longest, skinniest feet I have ever seen. The only major movement Fay made that day was to kick her legs. A vigorous, froglike movement that she still makes when she is happy. I like to think of it as her own version of leg pumping. Thinking of her little legs pumping underneath a smile marked by the gap between her two front teeth fills me with delight. She is her own person. And my delight in her is not diminished by my delight in her sister. I have called them by name. They are mine. They are precious and honored in my sight, and I love them . . . each in their own way.

3
Learning to Rest

"He rested from all the work
of creating that he had done."

GENESIS 2:3

MY FRIEND KATE RECENTLY GOT PREGNANT for the first time.

"How is Kate doing with the pregnancy?" I asked her husband.

Shaking his head in resignation he truthfully responded, "Well, you know, she thinks everything she does is indispensable. So she's having a really rough time."

I understood immediately. Women in my generation were fed ambition with our rice cereal. We have been told since birth that we can do anything we want to do and be anything we want to be. We have done our best to cash in on that promise. No job is too difficult. Cutting back on sleep is a small price to pay for achieving our dreams. There is no situation that a healthy dose of willpower and an unhealthy dose of caffeine can't solve.

For many of us, our dreams are not for ourselves. We dream of a better world. We work to help children, to build societies, to teach and feed and love those around us. But the altruism of our dreams does not dampen our ambition. In many cases, our altruism only fuels our willingness to give everything for the causes we have espoused.

Kate spends her working life between two jobs. She works with at-risk teens half the time. Then she works with families who have loved ones in prison. She spends her personal life with her five-year-old daughter whom they adopted a year ago. She spends the hours after her daughter is asleep visiting families and children for whom she has cared for many years. Kate was excited to get pregnant, but like the rest of us, she was not excited to have her energy cut in half.

We have a large glass window in our living room. I love it when my husband washes it. For the first few days I can barely tell there is even a window between me and the outside. Unfortunately, the birds can't tell there is a window there either. Every few weeks a resounding WHAM! echoes through the house, and I cringe as I open the door to see if the little feathered fellow made it through the crash.

I had been pregnant about one month. I wouldn't say I was quite soaring along. I had a strong case of morning sickness that was by no means limited to the mornings. But I sure didn't see the glass window coming. All of a sudden, I was slammed with exhaustion. I found myself lying on my bed, the couch, the floor of a friend's office, and any other available flat surface wondering what hit me.

"I think I have mono," I told my husband.

"You're just pregnant," he said. I cringed and wondered if I could take nine months of being so tired.

It's not that it's hard to be tired. There is nothing inherently hard about lying on the couch. There is nothing inherently hard about going to bed at eight (or seven!) o'clock. But giving up whatever it is you used to do before you slept so much? That's as hard as a plate glass window.

We've been taught that our self-worth is bound up with what we do. "What did you do today?" my mom asks each night when we talk on the phone. Her question stems from an interest in my life. But somehow, even as I approach thirty, I want to have something to report that will make her proud. I want to seem industrious and hardworking. I want my daily schedule to reflect my values. I hope that what I've done during the day has made a difference in the lives of others. Somehow, even knowing I was pregnant, I couldn't bring myself to answer, "Oh, you know, I slept in, did a little work, took a nap, did a little work, took another nap, and really I need to get off the phone cuz I'm planning to go to bed at 7:30." I was ashamed to be that person. I wondered what I was worth.

We act as though the work we do is the best reflection of who we are. When we meet new people, our first question after learning someone's name is, "What do you do?" We are known by our work. There is some good reason for this. What we do with our time does reflect what we value. This is why pregnancy's exhaustion is so difficult. The rest we must take and the new choices we must make about our quite limited time force us to reexamine our values.

I have always hated Sabbath. A day without work seems like a waste of time. Of course we need rest, but we have nighttime for that. And of course we need to take time to go to church and enjoy family, but why not get a little work done during those Sunday evening hours? Anyway, if I spread my work throughout the week, then I'll have moments to rest in each day. Why cram my work into six days so I can twiddle my thumbs in boredom on the seventh? Occasionally I have tried to practice something of a Sabbath. After all, the Bible is pretty clear that those who don't practice Sabbath should be put to death (Exod. 31:15, Exod. 35:2, Num. 15:32–36, you get the idea). But I never get very far. I feel like I am wasting my time. There is so much that needs doing in the world. Surely God would have us going about God's work.

In one of my attempts to honor the Sabbath, I read a book about it. The author suggested that there was an intimate relationship between the six days of work and the one day of rest. He even claimed that the days of work were all in service to the day of rest. The days of work led up to the day of rest. The days of work had no meaning without the day of rest. He was so excited about Sabbath that I really yearned to understand what he was saying. But I just couldn't. I had never experienced work that seemed to lead to rest. Like the rich young ruler, I went away from that book feeling sad, not knowing how to live into the joy the author was quite obviously experiencing.

Then I slammed into that window of pregnancy exhaustion. And even as I lay there reeling from the fall, I realized that for the first time in my life I was engaged in work that required rest. As I lay on my bed, trying to convince myself that it was okay to take two naps in one day, I thought about the passage on Sabbath that I had read so many years before. I was engaged in the work of creating new life. I was doing work that was like God's work. And for the first time in my life, I could imagine resting for a whole day, just like God did after creating the life of the world. The creative work was bound to the rest. The resting was a necessary part of the creating. One could not exist without the other.

But even as I came to embrace rest as necessary and a way to be like God, I still had to decide what to let go of. I still had to give up activities and cut back on time spent with those I love. I still had to make room for the rest I was coming to embrace. I had to decide what I valued most. More important, I had to decide what work God really wanted me to do and what work I needed to trust God to give to others.

Previously, I had assumed that Sabbath was about cramming everything I wanted to do in seven days into six days. The exhaustion of pregnancy made that impossible. I simply couldn't cram it all in. I learned out of necessity one of the lessons that Sabbath has to teach—that the work I have managed to accomplish in six days is enough. When we believe that everything we do is important, it is tempting to believe that we have to be the ones doing it. It is tempting to believe that if we don't do our good work, no one will, and God's world will be a worse place. It is tempting to believe that the salvation of the world (or at least our household) is dependent upon us.

Instead of doing everything that we think might be good and helpful in the world, we are forced to narrow our focus. In my limited time, I have to choose what to do. I have to ask, "What would God have me value most this day?" Sabbath rest and the rest of pregnancy teach us to believe that God is in control, that God can be trusted with the workings of our lives. In learning to give up some of the good things we want to do, we learn that even the things we are able to do are not necessary. They are a gift from God.

In chapter 18 of Matthew's Gospel, Jesus tells a story. He says:

"What do you think? If a man owns a hundred sheep, and one of them wanders away, will he not leave the ninety-nine on the hills and go to look for the one that wandered off? And if he finds it, truly I tell you, he is happier about that one sheep than about the ninety-nine that did not wander off. In the same way your Father in heaven is not willing that any of these little ones should be lost." (18:12–14)

I always thought it made more sense for the shepherd to stay and take care of the ninety-nine sheep, but during my pregnancy, God taught me to focus on one little lamb. As an ordained minister, having a child has felt like leaving a whole flock of sheep to care for one little baby. It doesn't always make sense to me. I wonder if it is the best use of my gifts. But I am convinced that this narrowing of focus to one little lamb is not simply a product of my own human limits; this narrowing of focus is an opportunity to experience and understand how God works.   ?

This parable claims that we worship a God who cares for little ones. This God will leave the bulk of God's loved ones to take care of a little lamb that gets lost. This doesn't make sense to me, but it is how God works. God chooses Abraham, one man out of many, and builds a special relationship with him. God makes him into the nation of Israel, and develops a special relationship with them. Jesus chooses twelve men out of all the crowds that follow him and invests the bulk of his ministry in just those twelve.

In each of these cases, God claims that the narrowing of focus will be a blessing to many. God tells Abraham, "I will bless you . . . and you will be a blessing. . . . All peoples on earth will be blessed through you" (Gen. 12:2–3). Jesus leaves his ministry with the eleven saying, "Go and make disciples of all nations, baptizing them in the name of the Father and of the Son and of the Holy Spirit, and teaching them to obey everything I have commanded you" (Matt. 28:19–20). We experience choosing one out of many as a loss. God knows it is a way to bless the world. God uses our exhaustion to teach us how to narrow our vision to the child growing within us. We are asked to believe that all the good work we give up in order to rest on one child's behalf will somehow be a blessing to all the peoples of the earth.

Our bodies force us into this lesson. Necessity can be a good teacher. But if we just rest out of necessity, we will miss the joy and mystery of Sabbath rest. In the Bible, the first mention of Sabbath after the creation story is in Exodus 16. The Israelites have just been freed from slavery under Pharaoh, and they are complaining about the dining options in the desert. "You should have left us in Egypt!" they gripe to Moses and Aaron. God responds by sending quail in the evenings and manna in the mornings. The Israelites are to gather only what they need for each day, but on the sixth day they are to gather two portions. On the seventh day they are to eat what they gathered the day before and enjoy a day of Sabbath rest.

On the seventh day, some of the people go out to gather manna anyway. In this story, it is pretty clear that the work of gathering food is completely dependent on God's prior gift. The Israelites' "work" is not primarily their own. And yet they still can't give it up. They are still tempted to go and gather. They, like us, cannot seem to let go of their own busy-ness. There is no manna to be found on the seventh day. The Israelites' work is in vain. The story ends like this:

> Then the LORD said to Moses, "How long will you refuse to keep my commands and my instructions? Bear in mind that the LORD has given you the Sabbath; that is why on the sixth day he gives you bread for two days. Everyone is to stay where they are on the seventh day; no one is to go out." So the people rested on the seventh day. (Exod. 16:28–30)

That last phrase is a direct parallel to the phrase from Genesis 2: "So on the seventh day God rested from all his work." But the refrain rings hollow in Exodus. The joy of God's rest in Genesis is gone. In Exodus, the people have done all they can to avoid Sabbath rest. They rest only after chastisement and command. They are compelled to rest.

Our pregnancy rest can be like this. We can rest only out of necessity. We can worry about what we are not doing. We can feel guilty and embarrassed about how much we sleep. We can try to work even when our bodies cry for us to do otherwise. Or we can rest like God does in Genesis. We can learn a Sabbath rest that God calls blessed and holy.

Isaiah 58 ends with these words:

> If you keep your feet from breaking the Sabbath
> and from doing as you please on my holy day,
> if you call the Sabbath a delight,
> and the LORD's day honorable,
> and if you honor it by not going your own way
> and not doing as you please or speaking idle words,
> then you will find your joy in the LORD. (58:13–14)

How do we move from accepting our need for rest to calling it a delight?

Around week seventeen I started to anticipate my baby's first kick. I read that I would be most likely to feel the baby kick if I had just eaten and was lying down, quiet and still, attuned to my body and my baby. So every evening after dinner, I would lay on the couch waiting for that first kick. Once the kicks became an hourly occurrence, I stopped my after-dinner ritual. Then, near the end of my pregnancy, I began it again. I had moved into my last weeks, and I was told I was supposed to monitor how much my baby kicked each day. Some days, when I was really busy, it seemed as if my child had not kicked at all. My midwife eased my fears about the baby's health by explaining that a child will often wait until a mother is still to really move. Our movement as mothers lulls our babies to sleep. When we stop, they have the freedom to move. She also told me that when I'm busy, I'm more likely to miss my child's movements.

The joy of feeling my child move within me required my stillness. Those times of lying still were not born of the necessity of exhaustion. I rested to deepen my communion with my child. I rested because resting allowed me to feel her presence within me.

Theologian Abraham Heschel writes of Sabbath, "It is a day on which we are called upon to share in what is eternal in time, to turn from the results of creation to the mystery of creation; from the world of creation to the creation of the world." Sabbath rest is a time to be still and feel the God within us. It is a time to turn from the work of our own hands to marvel at the work God is doing on our behalf.

We need time to meditate on the mystery of creation. In pregnancy, we are catapulted into profoundly God-like activity, and times of rest allow us to marvel at what we are doing with God. Times of stillness let our minds and spirits catch up with where our bodies are taking us.

"What are you doing?" asks my mom.

"I'm lying on the couch," I say, "and it is delightful, and blessed, and holy, and God-like to enjoy this sort of rest."

"Amen," agrees my mom.

4
The Work of Groaning

—

*"We know that the whole creation has been
groaning as in the pains of childbirth."*

ROMANS 8:22

I RECENTLY BOUGHT A MOTIVATIONAL CARD for a
friend who was graduating from a job skills program. The
card said in bright pink and purple letters:

> If you have a preference, voice it.
>
> If you have a question, ask it.
>
> If you want to cry, bawl.
>
> If you need help, raise your hand and
>
> jump up and down.

Perhaps you can now guess that I'm that person. I was
the one in second grade who waved her hand wildly with
the answer to a question, not quite understanding why the
teacher ever needed to hear anyone's voice besides my own.
Whenever I do the obligatory Myers-Briggs exercise during
team-building retreats, people are shocked to learn that
I'm an introvert. "But you talk so much!" they exclaim in

a surprised tone that I find more than mildly obnoxious. I talk during movies, yell when I'm mad, and squeal when food tastes really delicious or Christmas is less than a month away. I have trouble doing anything quietly.

I knew that labor would be no different. I knew well before I was ever pregnant that I might be the pregnant woman cursing her husband and vowing to never have sex again. It took only the smallest stretch of imagination to envision myself screaming with such force that foam flew out of my mouth at each contraction. My nosy neighbor sarcastically reports that when I went into labor with Naomi, he came over to see what natural birth was like, but stopped a block short of our house when he heard the noise I was making.

A few months into my first pregnancy, I was again reading one of my myriad birth books. Trying to be the exceptionally prepared mom, I was reading ahead in the section on labor and delivery. Wedged right between a paragraph about eating and techniques for using a birth ball was the horrifying news that yelling and screaming during labor can add to a laboring woman's tension and work against the contractions. My neurotic wheels immediately began turning, and I thought to myself that they should really tell that to people like me *before* we get pregnant, since people like me can obviously not give birth under oppressive conditions of silence. The news was so disturbing that I had to put it completely out of my mind. I told myself that

I would not let something so small as an incessant need to verbalize get in the way of a successful birth. I tucked this horrific news into the section of my brain where I catalogued all the things I planned to get to the bottom of during birthing class. Disaster was temporarily averted.

Dan and I took Bradley Method classes to prepare for Naomi's birth. Every Tuesday night for twelve weeks we drove some thirty minutes to sit with another expectant couple in the living room of a bubbly blond named Cherri. Cherri defied all stereotypes. She was an odd mix of cheerleader and football player, with broad shoulders, perfectly white teeth, and a no-nonsense attitude that was oddly sweet as tea. She was a typical suburban soccer mom who just happened to be adamant about natural childbirth. I often imagined her soundly beating the patookie out of anyone who threatened her children and then cheerfully offering them the Neosporin she kept in her purse for emergencies.

I loved Cherri. I had been worried that we might get some over-the-top, earth-mama hippie as our birth educator. I had braced myself for lectures about the possibility of pain-free birth. I cringed at the thought of someone serenely sitting in lotus pose describing how labor might be orgasmic. And I had to remind myself daily that I would not immediately walk out in protest if our educator told stories about the success of silent births. Clearly, I have problems with stereotyping. But Cherri defied every stereotype about natural childbirth that I could come up with. In doing so, she graciously gave me the space I needed to imagine my own grumpy, Advil-addicted, ready-to-scream-at-the-drop-of-a-hat self giving birth without the help of medication.

Cherri said all sorts of things that made me embarrassed. She said them matter-of-factly as if she were talking about the Dow Jones numbers for the day. She said them with her impish, cheerleader smile as if other people's husbands weren't even in the room. She said them every few minutes, barely giving me time to recover from the last embarrassing thing she said.

So maybe I was the only one embarrassed. We were, after all, talking about birth, a subject that inherently involves vaginas. And while I'm perfectly comfortable typing the word, I actually prefer not to say it out loud. Yes, you understand me correctly. And yes, you are remembering correctly that I have two little girls who of course have vaginas that need talking about. But I was taught and have continued to develop a veritable arsenal of suitable alternatives.

My discomfort with the word, however ridiculous, is deep-seated. I distinctly remember attending a church camp when I was thirteen years old. My best friend was fifteen, and her friends insisted that we sign up for the "Girls Only" break-out session. I had been eyeing the cake decorating and interpretive dance sessions, but being two years younger, I swallowed my insecurity and signed up with the older girls. The "Girls Only" session was a time to talk about, you guessed it, sex.

I'm sure the leaders had good reason for our opening exercise. We sat in a circle, some fifty giggling girls eager to at least *talk* about the forbidden fruit (since we'd all signed commitment cards the night before promising not to taste it). The two college-age women leading the group introduced our topic, explained that they knew the topic was awkward, and just as I was feeling like maybe these two understood how I was feeling, they explained that to get over this awkwardness, we were all going to yell, as loudly as we could, the word *vagina*. I felt cold sweat race out of my pores onto my new "Jesus Is Lord" T-shirt, and before I could decide how to politely excuse myself, I was surrounded by ecstatic screaming. I decided the best thing I could do was to open my mouth and pretend to yell with the boldness of my peers. As I silently mouthed the word I still hate to say, I vowed never to pass up an interpretive dance class again.

Yet there I was, sitting cross-legged in a much smaller, coed circle listening to a woman who talked for two hours each Tuesday night about what my vagina would be doing on the blessed day Naomi came into the world and what Dan and I could do to help accomplish the task.

One night we were talking about responses to the pain of contractions. What sorts of responses would help relax our pelvic floors and allow the contractions to do their work? What sorts of responses would increase our tension and work against the contractions? Cherri eventually came around to the topic of screaming, a seemingly natural response to a pain that made breaking my arm in high school seem quite tolerable. Just as I was bracing myself for the dreaded lecture on the positive attributes of silent births, Cherri surprised me with a delightful little truth.

"We don't make noise in labor because we're in pain," she said. "We groan because groaning helps us bring our children into the world."

Cherri went on to explain how high-pitched screams and yells do indeed add to the tension of a laboring woman. Such high-pitched screams fight against the contraction, deterring it from pulling open the cervix. The advocates of silent birth had that much right. But low-pitched groans do just the opposite. Moaning and groaning can actually help relax the pelvic floor and allow the contractions to do their work.

"If you want to make noise, opt for low moans and groans," Cherri pronounced assuredly. I felt a firm peace pushing the tension and worry out of my body. I felt my pelvic floor relax. I knew, deep inside myself, that I would groan during my contractions. My peace was temporarily rippled by Cherri's insistence that we practice groaning together and then watch a video of a laboring woman who had groaning down to an art. But I left the class holding the precious knowledge that my groans would not simply be a response to pain; my groans would actually help bring my baby into the world.

> We know that the whole creation has been groaning as in the pains of childbirth right up to the present time. Not only so, but we ourselves, who have the firstfruits of the Spirit, groan inwardly as we wait eagerly for our adoption to sonship, the redemption of our bodies. For in this hope we were saved. But hope that is seen is no hope at all. Who hopes for what they already have? But if we hope for what we do not yet have, we wait for it patiently. In the same way, the Spirit helps us in our weakness. We do not know what we ought to pray for, but the Spirit himself intercedes for us through wordless groans. (Rom. 8:22–26)

Romans 8 is all about groaning. Creation groans. We groan. The Spirit groans on our behalf. Romans 8 describes the frustration of living in the midst of suffering when we know God has something better in mind. Groaning is the response to frustration and suffering. Creation groans for all of the harm done to it by humans. Creation knows that God's children could do a better job of caring for the environment and longs for God's children to be revealed. Humans groan for the suffering and degradation of their bodies and eagerly expect a time when their bodies will be fully redeemed. The Spirit groans as she watches her children struggle along, not knowing how to pray for the abysmal situation in which they find themselves.

The groaning in Romans 8 is an expression of gut-wrenching suffering. But the groans of Romans 8 are more than a simple response to pain. The groans express a longing for something new. The groans accompany eager expectation for a time when we will fully become God's children. The Spirit's groans are intercessory prayer. Paul compares the groaning of creation to the groans of a mother in labor. In both cases, groaning brings together the pain of the present reality with hopeful struggle for new life. Groaning is work. It accomplishes something. Cherri knew what God has known for a long time: that groaning is a helpful tool for the hard, often discouraging work of bringing new life into the world.

I was in active labor with my second child for some twenty-four hours. I learned after her birth that she was "sunny-side up," an oddly cheerful description of an incredibly painful position. She came into the world with a lump on her head that was nearly the size of my fist. We would worry over that lump for the next two months as the blood in it slowly dissipated. During labor, babies have an instinct to tilt their heads back over and over again. If a child is facing the mother's spine, this instinct helps the baby move down the birth canal. Because Fay was backwards, her instinct caused her to bang her little head repeatedly against my pelvis.

Her instincts weren't serving either of us well. I would learn the details of what was happening inside my body after Fay was safely in my arms. But while I was stuck at nine centimeters for some four hours, I remember crying desperately to my birth team, "This just isn't working!" I choked out the words through a sticky mix of tears and sweat. Voicing my sense of futility felt like admitting defeat. But I was desperate for encouragement, for some new idea, for any way to move labor along and bring me and my child together in the way I knew we were meant to be. In Romans 8, Paul describes creation as "subjected to futility." My efforts at bringing Fay into the world felt futile.

My midwife suggested some new laboring positions, but she seemed most concerned that I had broken my pattern of low moans to scream out my frustration. She coached and encouraged me to resume those low tones. She said I was doing exactly what I needed to be doing. She said Fay would come in her own time. I felt the middle of my body tighten as the iron grip of another contraction took hold. I put my frustration aside and started a low moan. As the contraction built, my desperate longing for an end pushed its way into my weary conscience, and my moan turned into an angry groan. The contraction receded, leaving my wracked body still and silent against the side of the tub.

"Good work," said the midwife.

Groaning is good work. It is work that ushers in new life. Groaning is work that pregnant women learn well. Mothers don't just groan during labor. The nine months of pregnancy offered more opportunity than I wanted to practice the work of moaning and groaning. From low back pain to constipation, I learned to groan like a champ.

With a first child who came into the world at a whopping ten pounds and another arriving seventeen months later, I was diagnosed with "fatigued" stomach muscles during the last two months of my second pregnancy. Walking any further than the front porch sent lightning bolts of pain shooting through my abdomen. Support belts didn't come close to the kind of help my fatigued muscles needed. I ended up walking around for two months with a crib sheet tied around my stomach. Of course, someone else had to tie it on each morning and then again every few hours when it loosened. Between the discomfort of the sheet, the embarrassment of getting it on, and the lightning bolts of pain that made it through the jury-rigged contraption, I had groaning down to an art.

And my pregnancies were uncomplicated. I was never faced with any condition that seriously threatened my health or the health of my children. I never had to make decisions about whether my pregnancies should continue or be brought to an end. I never lost a child. In the grand scope of maternal groaning, I'm an amateur.

My friend Dayna is a pro.

My friends Eric and Dayna conceived their first child near the end of my second pregnancy. They had been trying for over a year and had recently begun fertility testing. The pregnancy came as an actively pursued surprise. Their family, church, and circle of friends joyously began planning showers, envisioning how to share child care responsibilities, and bugging the couple to start their Target registry. The baby's heartbeat was strong, and we were all looking forward to the twenty-week ultrasound when we would find out if this new little one was a girl or boy. The day of the ultrasound arrived. I went through the morning wondering when we would get the news. A little before noon, Eric called. His voice was tense.

"Something is seriously wrong," he said.

Later that day I learned from Dayna that she was carrying a little boy. Eric and Dayna named him Ethan. We learned that Ethan had a serious neural tube defect. He was missing a few of his organs and the back of his skull had never formed. Eric and Dayna were told that he may or may not live to term. Even if he made it through labor and delivery, Ethan would live for a few hours at most.

I chose my words carefully. "What are the next steps? I mean, will you have to go in for a procedure?" I asked the questions timidly. The words *abortion* or *D & C* seemed oddly inappropriate. How do you ask a mother when her dying child will die?

"We're not going to end the pregnancy," Dayna said. She spoke confidently. A note of grace and determination rang in her voice. Over the next five months I would grow accustomed to that tone. I would come to hear that mix of deep sorrow and determined hope as the voice of God. At the time, it was startling.

"Ethan has brought us so much joy. I love being his mom. I love providing a space for him to live. I want to do that for him until he dies naturally. I want to be his mom as long as I can." Dayna invited us to come and pray at their house that night.

That day began a season of groaning. We gathered together on couches and kitchen chairs to weep and groan to God. Eric and Dayna showed the remarkable grace of inviting others into their home to hear their groans and join with them. They groaned together and groaned alone. They prayed when it made sense, and they were honest that sometimes prayer made no sense at all. In those honest moments, the Spirit groaned on their behalf.

They learned to groan and enjoy Ethan at the same time. They cherished his movements. Dayna would quickly bring

Eric's hand to her belly every time Ethan kicked. I would watch them stop whatever they were doing to turn toward their son until his movements stopped. They didn't want to miss a moment of time with him. They showered love on their little unseen son with care that put my parenting to shame.

The rest of us wanted to pray for Ethan's healing. We wanted to lament Ethan's defect. We wanted to name what was happening as a tragedy. We wanted to tell God it was unfair. Eric and Dayna patiently explained that those things weren't helping. They asked instead that we help them find ways to celebrate Ethan's life. They asked for help in holding together the dueling realities of Ethan's life and death.

So we rented them a handheld Doppler, and they listened to Ethan's heartbeat as if the music of his life rivaled Eric's beloved jazz tunes. They cancelled their Target registry, and we made donations to a prenatal hospice program in honor of Ethan's life. We planned a prayer shower to celebrate Ethan while showering the couple with the prayer they would need to weather the birth and death of their first child.

Eric and Dayna taught us the truth of biblical groaning. They taught us the truth that we are called to lament death and cherish life at exactly the same time. Dayna's groans were a place where gut-wrenching pain and hope for new life held together. Her groaning was beautiful. And completely confounding. I simply don't know how she did it. As one who was nearly undone by fatigued stomach muscles, I can't imagine being a mother so full of grace.

Ethan was born a few weeks before his due date. He lived for a few hours. For every minute of those hours he was held in the warm cradle of his parents' hands. He wore one of the fifteen caps his grandmother had knit for him. Not knowing when he would be born, she had diligently knit a cap each week, slightly increasing the size each time.

When I arrived at the hospital, Ethan was still there with his parents. I had the honor of holding him so they could eat chicken pad thai from the noodle bar next to the hospital. I laughed with Eric and Dayna about how Ethan's feet were as long and skinny as Eric's. I felt the impossible softness of his skin as it grew cold in my hands. My body rocked slightly as I held him, a habit I picked up to soothe my own girls. When I realized what I was doing, my spirit groaned. The tears that had been hovering so long at the edges of my eyes spilled over. I still feel dizzy thinking about it.

Ethan's funeral continued to hold together life and death, celebration and mourning. We watched a video of pictures taken at Ethan's birth. We practiced the groaning we had learned so well. Eric's father read a passage from Isaiah 65. The passage, like Romans 8, expresses a deep longing for a new creation, for a time when death and suffering will be no more. Eric's father slowly climbed the stairs leading to the altar, the maroon carpet padding what appeared to be incredibly difficult steps. He opened his Bible and read,

> See, I will create
> new heavens and a new earth.
> The former things will not be remembered,
> nor will they come to mind.
> But be glad and rejoice forever
> in what I will create,
> for I will create Jerusalem to be a delight
> and its people a joy.
> I will rejoice over Jerusalem
> and take delight in my people;
> the sound of weeping and of crying
> will be heard in it no more.
> Never again will there be in it
> an infant who lives but a few days. . . .
> They will not labor in vain
> nor will they bear children doomed to misfortune;
> for they will be a people blessed by the LORD.
> (Isa. 65:17–20, 23)

From where I was sitting I could see Dayna lean her head against Eric's shoulder. I held my own little girl tight. I wanted to yell. I wanted to hurl hymnals at the altar. I wanted to scream, "This isn't working!" But all I could manage was a little moan. Maybe a low moan was just what the situation needed. My daughter looked at me and rubbed my chest with her toddler hands. She seemed to have Dayna's gift for holding together life and death.

Groaning is hard and exhausting work. Most godly work is. When my groaning finally brought Fay into the world, I was shaking and nauseated. I felt like I had been run over by a truck. Not in a rush-her-to-the-ER sort of way. I felt like one of those frogs who has been run over so many times for so many days by so many trucks that she is thin, flat, and entirely dried up. I felt like a crispy, thin, sun-dried frog. My throat was sore from the groaning.

Dayna now smiles a tired, knowing smile from behind her wire-rimmed glasses. Her tall, thin frame leans back a bit when she talks to me, as if to narrow the difference in our heights. She has stick-straight, white-blond hair, and I'm quite certain God meant for us to notice that when Dayna stands in the sun her hair glows like the golden rings we paint around the heads of Mary and Jesus. Maybe she feels like a sun-dried frog too, but she looks to me like the face of God.

PART TWO
Bearing the Marks of Christ

5
Redefining Attractive

"His face shown like the sun."

MATTHEW 17:2

"YOU'RE PREGNANT! IT'S THE ONLY TIME in your life you can be fat and feel good about it!" I had said it to others, and now it was payback time. When I tried to share with friends and family my growing discomfort about my growing size, I was met with some variation of the above saying. There is a kernel of truth in the saying. There are ways that the "rules" about what is attractive and what is not change during pregnancy. I was encouraged to eat that second piece of pie for which a nonpregnant woman would have been scolded (or at least talked about). Weight gain (especially if limited to one's midsection) is considered a positive accomplishment. And the swelling breasts and bellies of pregnant women have long been the subject of many an artist.

But for most of the eighteen months I have spent pregnant, I have not felt beautiful. I have not been comfortable with my growing size. I have not believed for a minute that being pregnant somehow transforms varicose veins into a lovely thing. I have had difficulty convincing myself that being attractive means something totally different than what I have known it to mean all my life. From what I've heard from the women around me, I'm not alone.

We women spend some fifteen to forty years of our lives learning the rules of the game. Attractive equals tall, thin, a clear complexion, a flat stomach, great hair, and the like. All of a sudden we find ourselves thicker than ever, retaining water, splotchy, veiny, stretch-marked, enlarging in the middle, and to top it all off, a dark line is beginning to descend from our belly buttons (which are no longer cute and pierce-able but appear to be on the verge of exploding). We're told we don't have to play by the "normal" rules, but we aren't told what the new rules are.

It doesn't help that all the models in the maternity section are still playing by the old rules. I remember standing in a big box store trying to figure out where the maternity section was. I stood in front of a life-size glossy image of a classic blond. Her long hair flowed across a perky chest. She looked like she was walking with a bouncy step. Her pearly white smile suggested that she'd had a perfect morning, or at least hadn't spent the morning bent over the toilet. The only thing that suggested the possibility of pregnancy was the empire waist on her shirt. I couldn't even make out a real bump below the seam. As it turned out, this woman did indeed represent the maternity section, but it took me inspecting numerous other images and finding the "Maternity" sign to figure that out.

Was I supposed to look like that model? What does it mean to be attractive while pregnant? Can we make ourselves more attractive? Where is God in all of this? For me, the journey through some of these questions began in the grocery store line.

I am not a "touchy" person. I dread passing the peace at church. I always feel slightly offended that the preacher would interrupt a perfectly good service and unabashedly ask me to leave the comfort of my well-chosen, back-row pew to brave a deluge of hugs and handshakes. Truth be told, it actually takes a great deal of energy for me to hug even those I love most. So you can imagine my horror when I finally began to "look pregnant" with my first child. Almost overnight, around month six, I went from looking possibly pregnant to looking classically pregnant. And with that change, strangers went from lobbing hesitant, questioning smiles directed at my midsection to full-on touch.

Women at my church, in my family, and even at work thought nothing of plopping their hands directly on my belly without even giving me a proper greeting. Going to the grocery store became an exhausting social excursion. Even the occasional bold man would give his least creepy smile and ask permission to "feel the baby." I was touched by so many people that I even began noticing a few different categories of touch.

There was the one-handed, light, "I know I shouldn't be doing this but I just have to get in one little touch" touch. This touch was delivered briskly, almost as if testing a stove burner for heat. This touch often came accompanied by a shy smile and apology (after the fact) for the imposition.

There was the two-handed "assessment" touch. This was almost exclusively delivered by middle-aged women, long-time moms, and those on the verge of becoming grandmothers. One of my least favorite touches, it normally involved numerous hand placements, as if the woman was assessing a watermelon. I also disliked this touch for the comments that ensued. "Whoa, you're huge!" "Hmmm . . . carrying high, I see!" Nothing in my past had prepared me for such public assessment of my figure.

There was the exploratory "find the baby" touch, mostly executed by health care providers, my mother, and one particular aunt. Thankfully, this sort of deep (often painful) probing occurred in relative private by those who felt particularly assured in their claims on my body. I didn't mind this touch quite as much as the others as it normally yielded some new, highly coveted bit of information about my growing baby.

And then there was the rub. Round, massaging circles accompanied by coos of, "Oh, I just *love* pregnant bellies!" At the beginning of this phenomenon, I tried to smile politely at the rubbers, feeling sure this was the socially appropriate response. By the end of my pregnancy, I realized that they were so lost in the joy of rubbing a pregnant belly that I really didn't have to hide my disdain; they almost never looked at my face.

Those who couldn't bring themselves to touch stared. Even the staring baffled me. "Don't stare," my mother repeated throughout my childhood. "It's rude." And yet people who I am certain received the same cultural training stared without restraint. They stared with a sort of starry-eyed reminiscence. They stared in an awestruck, I-can't-help-but-stare sort of way. They stared with proud congratulations.

And the stare-ers and the touch-ers all shared their stories. The check-out line at the grocery store seemed to particularly invite these stories. Never in my previous life could I recall having spoken to anyone at all in the check-out line (recall, I'm an introvert). Now I was a veritable talk show host. I heard stories about grandchildren just born. I heard stories about how difficult the wife's second pregnancy had been. I heard stories about how women carried "low just like that" when they had boys. And I answered questions. How far along? Boy or girl? First child? Have you thought of a name?

I considered asking people to stop. I considered avoiding the conversations or sending my husband to the grocery store. But the Southern-woman training I can't seem to get out of my head said that would be impolite. And then, quite unexpectedly, this touching and talking began to change me. I noticed a shift in the way I thought about this interest in my body. While I began with an appalled, "Why do they think they can touch me!?" by month seven I found myself pondering the situation with a half-smile.

"Huh, they want to touch me," I'd think. By month eight, while the touching was still uncomfortable, I found myself thinking with a full smile, "That's sort of cool—strangers want to touch me." And by month nine, I'd begun to ponder in my heart a curious and delightful thought—strangers wanted to touch Jesus too.

The Bible tells of many times in which crowds gather around Jesus. Zacchaeus climbs a tree just to look at this teacher. Occasionally the crowd pressed in so close that Jesus would retreat, either to solitude or to the sea. Luke tells the story of when a woman who had bled for twelve years touched Jesus.

As Jesus was on his way, the crowds almost crushed him. And a woman was there who had been subject to bleeding for twelve years, but no one could heal her. She came up behind him and touched the edge of his cloak, and immediately her bleeding stopped.

"Who touched me?" Jesus asked.

When they all denied it, Peter said, "Master, the people are crowding and pressing against you."

But Jesus said, "Someone touched me; I know that power has gone out from me." (Lk. 8:42–46)

So many people have touched Jesus that the disciples wonder at his question. We can imagine Peter rolling his eyes and muttering, "Who *hasn't* touched you?" But even though Jesus has been touched by so many, he is still attuned to the unique circumstances that draw each individual person to his body. Jesus has been touched a million times, but this one person who touched him still matters in all of her individuality.

Not only is Jesus willing to be touched, he also wants to look into the faces of those who touch him. He doesn't want to be touched like some sort of good luck charm. He wants to hear the stories of those who seek healing. Jesus knows that power has gone out of him. He could have left it at that. But Jesus seeks out conversation with the one who has experienced the power of touching him. The woman who touched him can't turn down his invitation. She comes trembling and kneels before him (somewhat like the timid tummy-touchers with their retroactive apologies!). She tells him her story. She tells what touching him meant to her. He tells her to "go in peace."

As I pondered this story, I was amazed at the similarities between Jesus' situation and my own. Jesus can hardly go anywhere in public without being touched. Those touches, like the ones in the grocery store line, open the way for people to share their stories with Jesus. The stories are quite personal, often involving life histories of pain, sickness, and hopelessness. Jesus shares this intimate moment with the one who touches him and then the two part ways.

But for all the similarities, there was one glaring difference. Jesus knew his own power. When Jesus is touched, he knows immediately that power has gone out of him. Does my body have power like that? Power to heal? I still find the thought alternately scary and laughable.

I was visiting with a woman my age and her mother. The woman was not much more than an acquaintance, but I knew she had been trying to get pregnant for some time. We had crossed paths while I was taking a walk, and as we ended our brief conversation, the mother said to her daughter, "Well, you better rub her belly before we go. Help you get pregnant, you know." The daughter looked embarrassed but timidly reached out to fulfill what clearly had been intended as a command, and the two walked on. I couldn't move from the spot. I couldn't imagine anyone ascribing such power to my tummy.

I marveled at this event for weeks. And then, much to my surprise, it happened again! And again. A hefty handful of times throughout my two pregnancies I have been confronted with this particular tidbit of folklore. And each time I have smiled politely and prayed quietly as some hopeful mother-to-be reached out to touch me and the growing baby inside me.

I do not know the origin of this particular old wives' tale. I cannot testify to its truth. But I have come to believe that the old wives who tell it know something I am slow to admit— that pregnant women do have a certain, undeniable power. A power to heal. A power to bring smiles. A power to invite conversation and relationship where no such opportunity existed before. These old wives know that pregnant women, like Jesus, are attractive.

Pregnant women are attractive in that they draw others to themselves. Pregnant bellies have a power to invite touch, to welcome stories, to open the possibility for relationship. Cultivating this kind of beauty is not a question of hairstyles, make-up, or what type of dress might possibly hide the fact that I've become as big as a whale. Cultivating this kind of beauty means asking, "How can I better welcome those who are attracted to me? How can I, like Jesus, invite their stories? How can I, like Jesus, see the specific needs and joys of each person who comes? How can I, like Jesus, bless the tummy-touchers and send them in peace, even when I feel almost crushed by the crowds? How can I, like Jesus, know and rest in my own power to attract and to heal?"

Pregnant women teach us that attraction is not primarily about how we look, but about how well we attract others to ourselves and how well we welcome them once they draw near.

I believe that. With all my heart. But I have to confess that, at the end of the day, I still want to *look* pretty. There, I've said it. Attracting others to myself is all fine and good. It is an amazing, holy mystery in which I get to be like Jesus. *AND* . . . I still want to look pretty. I want to be attractive in the Jesus way and in the head-turning, did-you-see-her way too. And I've begun to think that God doesn't see my desire to look pretty as completely unholy.

I worked as a teaching assistant in seminary when I was pregnant with my first child. Many times in my first trimester I ducked out of class to race to the bathroom, praying desperately that God might enable me to throw up in a socially acceptable place like the toilet. I hate throwing up, and I remember walking back through the empty halls disgusted and annoyed. On one such return, an older student emerged from a neighboring classroom. She looked at me, and her face broke into a smile.

"You're glowing!" she exclaimed.

"You're kidding," I thought.

The glow of pregnancy is an incomprehensible phenomenon to me. Without fail, when I was feeling my most tired, most disgusting, most bloated, someone would look at me as if seeing me for the first time and joyously proclaim, "You're glowing!" It was inconceivable, and I loved it. I would push my disbelief just slightly to the side and bask in the compliment.

The truth is, while pregnant women redefine *attractive* as an ability to attract others to themselves, they also redefine *pretty*. Pregnant bodies insist on their own beauty, even when it fails to meet any conventional standards. "I may have swollen ankles, I may fit into none of my clothes, I may have red blotches on my face, but I can glow!" our pregnant bodies shout. "Did you hear me? I can glow!" our bodies shout louder in the face of our own disbelief. And the remarkable truth is that this startling, quite physical beauty is Christ-like too. The glow of pregnancy is not a glow one can salt-scrub into existence. It is instead a beauty that overflows from the welcome a pregnant woman offers to her baby and to those who are attracted to her. The glow of pregnancy is the glow that comes from being in the presence of God and being involved in God's activity.

Jesus glowed with this sort of beauty. Matthew 17 tells the story of when Jesus brought his best friends with him to the top of a mountain. Matthew writes, "There [Jesus] was transfigured before them. His face shown like the sun, and his clothes became as white as the light" (17:2). Jesus glows at an important point in his ministry. He is moving steadily toward the cross and has just explained his own death to his disciples. He has just told them that they too must suffer if they are to follow in his footsteps. The change in Jesus' physical appearance marks a change in his orientation. As he begins to prepare for his suffering and death, his face begins to glow. Perhaps the glow of pregnancy is like the glow of Jesus: it attends those who are willing to suffer to bring new life to others.

Jesus also glowed because he was in the presence of God. Moses glowed this way too. Moses went up to Mount Sinai to talk face-to-face with God. When he came down the mountain, carrying the laws that God had given, Exodus tells us, "His face was radiant because he had spoken with the LORD" (34:29). But Moses didn't know his face was glowing. He had to be told. Like the pregnant woman who feels her least attractive, Moses was completely unaware of the startling physical beauty that comes from being in the presence of God. I can almost imagine Moses' incredulous response to being told of his glow. "I'm what? Glowing? Well, Aaron, if you say so . . . "

The truth is, doing God's work is hard. We imagine being in God's presence as something sublime. We imagine beauty in the same way. Both should feel good. But being in God's presence is difficult. Doing God's work requires sacrifice and a willingness to suffer. It requires that we orient our lives to the needs of others. It rarely feels sublime, and we don't imagine ourselves looking pretty while we do it. And yet Jesus, Moses, and pregnant women glow. They take up the work of the cross, they enter the presence of God, they partner with God in God's work, and they glow. They glow with a startling, physical beauty.

I don't know that I could have made it up Mount Sinai when I was pregnant, even if a face-to-face with God was the prize at the end of the hike. But if I did, I imagine God would have said something like this to my sweaty, overexerted face:

"I want you to know how attractive you are . . . so watch out! You'll be so attractive you won't know what to do with all the people who want to touch you. What I'd like you to do is welcome them. Hear their stories. Send them in peace. As for beauty, you'll glow as one who has been in my presence. It won't feel like going to the spa, more like going to the cross, but you'll shine like the sun. Enjoy it, and try to remember what being attractive is really about, even after you give birth."

6
Suffering and New Life

"I bear on my body the marks of Jesus."

GALATIANS 6:17

MY FRIEND AMY LAURA HAS A MINI-FUTON in her office. It is covered by a bold, multicolored quilt that a number of her students knit together while listening to her lectures. I was lying on top of the futon with my hands tucked underneath. I couldn't seem to get them far enough from my nose to stop the nausea.

"My own hands are making me sick!" I sobbed out the words. I was completely defeated.

For the last two months I had grown accustomed to throwing up each day. I had learned to avoid the smell of coffee, cooking onions, malls, and anything that might make an appearance at the state fair. I had tried to gracefully accept that those smells would send me hurtling to the nearest bathroom, bag, or shrub. I understood that part of being pregnant was a heightened sense of smell, and part of me being pregnant was nausea related to about half of the new smells I was smelling.

But now my hands were making me sick, and I couldn't do a thing about it. I could not avoid them or easily detach them. As I lay on Amy Laura's couch with hair and dried vomit stuck to my face, I seriously considered cutting them off. Thankfully, Amy Laura suggested a very potent mint lotion. I had my doubts that anything could cover up the smell of garlic that had been embedded in my fingertips during an ill-planned cooking extravaganza the night before. I had scrubbed them and applied all the lotion in my bathroom, purse, and hotel mini-bottle collection. I had rubbed my hands on stainless steel, an old trick for removing the smell of garlic and onions that had worked in the past but refused to work at this crucial moment. But Amy Laura dug through a pile of books, some dusty icons, and a few of her children's finger paintings to produce the most pungent lotion I have ever smelled. For a moment, I was afraid that the smell of the lotion would be worse than the garlic, but as the smell of fresh-picked peppermint filled the room, I felt my nausea slowly back down.

I was completely unprepared for the nausea I felt during pregnancy. I get motion sick in cars, planes, boats, trains, merry-go-rounds, and golf carts that don't go fast enough. I pride myself on having learned to adapt to this sickness, and I figured I would be well prepared for the nausea of pregnancy. I had never heard any truly horrific stories about morning sickness. I had even heard some encouraging ones about women who threw up in their trashcans and went straight to board meetings in the next room.

"Some women don't even get morning sickness," my mom had said.

But as soon as I found myself daily scrubbing the toilet in preparation for the inevitable moment when I would place my head on it, the horror stories came rolling in. It was as if my first vomit inducted me into some secret women's society. Women who had never before said an unpleasant word in my presence broke their perfectly lipsticked smiles to share the most shocking pregnancy-related stories.

"Well, you know Ms. Barbara had to be hospitalized three times for dehydration due to vomiting," said one woman from my church.

"And Susan's nausea never once stopped. I heard she threw up every day of those nine months," said another.

"Well, I was on bed rest the last three months of my second pregnancy, and taking care of a one-year-old all the while," chimed in a third.

I was certain these same women had called pregnancy a blessing. I had watched them give birth to child after child. I couldn't remember ever having heard them previously complain about anything more serious than the wrong flowers being chosen for the mission-banquet centerpiece. But as I vomited my way through my first months of pregnancy, their stories of hospitalizations, back pain, thirty-hour labors, and third-degree tears came rolling in. On the day when my constipation became so severe that I had to wrap my hand in toilet paper and physically pull my own poop out of my behind, I vowed to be honest about the crap of pregnancy *before* the women around me started throwing up.

The truth is, pregnancy hurts. Of course, there are those women who insist on gushing obnoxious phrases like, "I just *love* being pregnant!" There are those women who don't get morning sickness . . . ever. But most women, even the ones who never throw up, experience some sort of suffering at some point during their pregnancies.

Historically, even death was a real possibility during childbirth. In many developing countries, it still is. While most of us have access to prenatal care and well-resourced delivery rooms, Amnesty International produced a report in 2010 exposing the maternal death rate in the United States. Even though the United States spends more than any other nation on maternal health care, we rank below forty other countries in the number of women that we let die in childbirth. We have the resources to prevent most maternal deaths in our country, but many women are denied access to those resources. African American women are four times more likely to die in childbirth than white women in the United States. Death in childbirth is not so far in the past as we might like to think.

As I began thinking about the Christian significance of pregnancy, I searched the Bible for references to childbirth and labor. I had some vague memories of the Bible imaging God as a brooding mother hen, and I remembered something about a rock who labored to give birth to Israel. I felt sure the Bible must be filled with more such images of God as a laboring woman. To my horror, most of the references to labor were paired with the word *pain*. As in, "She was overcome by her labor pains." This was 1 Samuel's polite way of describing the death of Phinehas' wife. When God is imaged as a laboring woman in Isaiah, the description goes something like, "For a long time I have kept silent, I have been quiet and held myself back. But now, like a woman in childbirth, I cry out, I gasp and pant." God goes on to nearly destroy Israel in this passage, as a sort of macabre mother-gone-wild. The Israelites are described as laboring women when they are being destroyed in battle. In short, when the Bible imagines labor, the Bible imagines panting, pain, and death close behind.

Even if we take death off the table, even if we get an epidural before a planned induction, even if we try self-hypnosis for a pain-free birth, we must face that part of pregnancy is learning to suffer. Part of pregnancy is learning to look death in the face. As my childbirth educator put it, "Pregnancy is about embracing not just any pain, but pain for a purpose."

I sat at the tiny, round tea table that my friend Thea had managed to squeeze into her crowded office. Thea had been my professor in seminary. She had taught me Hebrew and directed my thesis. She is one of those rare, somewhat scary people who begins sentences with absurd phrases like, "Last night before I went to bed I was perusing a sixteenth-century Greek grammar book, and I noticed . . . " After a handful of such sentences, I developed a deep respect, hidden love, and healthy fear of this intense professor. But the day I sat at her tiny tea table, I was no longer a student. Our relationship was transitioning to friendship, and I had come to tell her I was pregnant. She asked all the right questions about due dates and where I would have the baby. I asked her where she had given birth to her son and whether or not she had gotten an epidural. Her happy I'm-glad-you're-pregnant smile dropped.

"My situation was sort of complicated," she said. Her eyes squinted a bit, the way they do when she is deciding how to word something. I sat quietly, trying not to look too eager, so she could decide how much of her story she wanted to tell. I guess she decided she could trust me. A deeply peaceful smile started in her eyes and began to inch out from behind her serious semifrown. As she slowly began the story of her pregnancy and labor, I knew that I was officially transitioning from student to friend. That day, at the tea table covered in embroidered purple cloth, Thea told me how her only child came into the world.

When she got pregnant, Thea was a busy and ambitious graduate student with precise plans for how her baby might be neatly tucked between classes and dissertation writing. Things were going according to plan until her last trimester. Then, well before her baby could live outside of her womb, Thea's body began to labor. She was immediately hospitalized. She was placed on muscle relaxers to stop the contractions. The medicine worked for a while, but her body fought back, determined to have its way. As Thea's contractions became stronger, she was given more and more muscle relaxers.

"By the end, the medicine was so strong that I couldn't move! Literally, from the neck down, I was immobile!" She laughed a kind of hysterical laugh. It's the kind of laugh you laugh when something is so absurd, even ten years later, that you either have to laugh or cry. She described lying for weeks on that hospital bed, completely immobile and dependent, robbed of everything that had formerly given her life meaning.

Before being hospitalized, Thea filled her days with work that gave her life purpose. Whether it was teaching, writing, or investing in relationships, Thea was busily and actively engaged in activity that she could feel good about. The medications to prevent Sebastian's early labor took all of those activities from her. But as she lay on that hospital bed, Thea began to realize that her life was taking on a different sort of meaning.

I watched the light stream in behind her through leafy trees and a wall-sized gothic window. The light bounced off her hair as she explained how she felt. "My whole purpose in life was to bring that child into the world," she said. "I didn't know if I would live, but if I could give life to Sebastian, that would be enough. For the first time, I knew what it meant to give my life for someone else."

I don't remember anything she said after that. I don't remember how long we talked, or what I said, or when I left. Because at that moment I looked at her and saw someone who had given up life as she knew it to give life to another human being. I looked at her and knew I was looking at Jesus. She might as well have shown me the marks in her hands and side.

I wanted to tell her what I saw in her, to tell her that the Jesus in her was glowing. But, let's face it, if you say that in your first "friend conversation" with someone, you'll likely not be invited back for a second. So I squeezed my enthusiasm into the back of my throat and concentrated on not crying while she finished her story.

Thea had given over her life and accepted the possibility of her death to bring Sebastian into the world. She had been Christ to him. And while the details of her particular story make it easy to see Jesus shining through, every pregnant woman makes something of this sacrifice. Every pregnant woman is willing to suffer to bring new life into the world.

At the heart of the Christian faith is the affirmation that Jesus' suffering, death, and resurrection break open the possibility for our new life. For the Apostle Paul, being a Christian meant taking Jesus' death and resurrection into his own body. As he was persecuted for preaching the gospel, Paul understood his suffering to mirror the suffering of Christ. Because Jesus had lived on the other side of suffering and death, Paul knew he would too. Paul understood baptism as a mirror of Christ's death and being raised out of the waters as joining in the resurrection of Jesus. Paul explained that when we give up sin, we die to the world. When we choose a new sort of lifestyle, we join in the new life of Christ. For Paul, Jesus' suffering, death, and resurrection are the basic pattern of life. Paul looks around and sees the pattern everywhere.

At the end of his letter to the Galatians, Paul takes the pen from his scribe to write to his friends in his own hand. He ends the letter by saying, "I bear on my body the marks of Jesus" (Gal. 6:17). It is the last and most important thing he can think to say. If they miss everything else, he wants them to see in his large and scrawling print the heart of his message: "I bear in my body the marks of Jesus."

We can go overboard seeing the pattern of Jesus' life and death all around us. As an insightful friend once said, "Every splinter in the road is not the cross." Some suffering is just wrong. Some suffering must be denounced and should be avoided. Jesus incessantly spoke out against the suffering of the poor and infirm and eased their suffering when he could. Sometimes suffering comes to us because of what we believe, but we discern that it isn't our time to go to the cross. After all, Jesus miraculously slipped through angry mobs a number of times before he was crucified.

But every once in a while, we come upon suffering that mirrors the suffering of Christ. We come upon suffering that can help usher new life into the world. As Christians, we are sometimes given the gift of bearing that kind of suffering ourselves. And in those moments, we become the mirror image of Jesus. We, like Paul, bear in our bodies the marks of Christ.

Pregnancy and labor offer just this sort of opportunity. One night in my birthing class we talked about the pain of labor. Cherri called it "pain for a purpose," and she explained that knowing your pain is for a purpose makes all the difference in how you experience that pain. Pain can wear away at your soul. Anyone who has experience with terminal illness knows this truth. Pain like that accomplishes nothing but the further deterioration of our precious bodies. But the pain of labor is different. The pain of labor promises to bring new life into the world. A woman's body breaks open, not to accomplish her death, but to create new life. Death is a possibility. But death is not the purpose.

I don't like the way life and death come together at the cross. I don't know why new life should come out of death.

It seems that God, being God and all, could have just brought forth the new life part without the suffering and death part. I don't like the way life and death come together in pregnancy either. It just doesn't make sense that the blessing of a new baby should come through so much pain. I don't think I'm alone in being bothered by this pairing of suffering and new life. The writers of Scripture find the pain of labor so troubling that they include an explanation within the first three chapters of the Bible! They can't imagine labor pains as part of God's original plan, so they explain the pain of labor as Eve's punishment for eating of the tree of the knowledge of good and evil.

But as much as I hate it, suffering and new life are welded together by God on the cross. It is the mystery at the heart of my faith. And even though it seems like a curse, pregnant women bring this same sort of suffering into themselves every time a child is born. As a pregnant woman breaks open in labor, the blood and water that pour from her are perhaps as close as we will ever come to witnessing the blood and water that poured from Jesus' side on the cross. Curse becomes the blessing of new life, by God's grace and one servant's suffering.

My housemate Jonathan used to make delicious tomato soup with big chunks of tomato floating in it. We ate the soup with greasy grilled-cheese sandwiches. During the winter months, it was a standard meal.

He made this soup one unfortunate day in mid-November when I was pregnant with Naomi. I smelled the soup as soon as I walked into the kitchen and knew, without a doubt, that I shouldn't eat it. But it was my first pregnancy, and I was still learning how to politely reject other people's cooking. I threw up way less during my second pregnancy. I attribute this entirely to the fact that I was then a seasoned pregnant mom who had learned how to say, "That looks just lovely, but I'm so nauseous right now I don't think I should try any." But on that night in mid-November, I had not yet learned the art of politely declining food, so I girded up my loins and faced the soup whose smell was turning me a pale shade of green.

We all sat down to dinner. I quietly sipped my soup. I swallowed a few of the tomatoes. I tried to smile sweetly as I whispered to my husband, "I'm going to be sick." And then I folded my napkin neatly in my chair before rushing off to the bathroom. It was the worst bout of vomiting I've ever experienced. The three tomato chunks I had managed to get down came back out through my nose. I'm quite certain you could hear the reappearance of the tomato chunks back at the dinner table because Jonathan has not made his signature soup in the four years since.

I'm not sure that vomiting tomato chunks through my nose counts as taking up the cross. Perhaps that is one of the splinters along the road to which my insightful friend was referring. But I do know that it hurt like hell. I also know that the hormones that made me throw up that day were hormones that made it possible for my baby to live within my body. Perhaps throwing up through one's nose is the lightest form of suffering. But it is a suffering that is mysteriously connected to bringing new life into the world.

I know it's not polite to talk about tomato chunks coming out of my nose or pulling a turd from my behind. I've had to give my good, Southern-woman upbringing five or six valiums just to get the facts down on paper. But I've decided that silence about the suffering of pregnancy just doesn't help. I think there is some fear that telling the full truth about pregnancy will be too discouraging to mothers-to-be. We fear that if we talk about suffering, no one will ever become a mother again. But the truth is, no suffering in the world could have kept me from having my babies. Naming my suffering has helped me learn my own strength. Naming the suffering of others has helped me see Christ in them. Telling the truth, even about "indecent" bodily functions, is important, faithful work.

I found the story of Rachel's death when I was in seminary. It was tucked quietly into Genesis 35, between God reaffirming the covenant with Jacob and a list of the twelve tribes. The whole story is only five verses long. Her death is also the story of Benjamin's birth.

Rachel was the love of Jacob's life. I had learned in Sunday school how Jacob had worked for seven years to marry Rachel but had been tricked into marrying her older sister, Leah. Jacob worked another seven years to win Rachel for a wife as well. My fifth-grade heart would swoon at the story. It was the closest thing to Disney that we got on Sunday mornings.

As the Bible tells it, God looks down on Leah and sees how painful it would be to be an unloved older sister. God opens her womb, and Leah gives birth to son after son. Rachel, the favored one, struggles to have any children at all. Finally, Rachel gives birth to Joseph, and he is his father's favorite son. And then, just when the family story seems to be coming to a close, Rachel becomes pregnant again. She bears the last of Jacob's sons, the twelfth tribe of Israel. Genesis 35 tells the story of the birth. The text says:

> Rachel began to give birth and had great difficulty. And as she was having great difficulty in childbirth, the midwife said to her, "Don't despair, for you have another son." As she breathed her last—for she was dying—she named her son Ben-Oni. But his father named him Benjamin. (35:16–18)

With her dying words, Rachel names the son for whom she dies. She calls him Ben-Oni. The name means "son of my suffering." His name would have told the story of the life she gave for him. But his father calls him Benjamin. It means "son of my right hand." The right hand was the hand of power and favor. Benjamin is a strong, triumphant, and powerful name. It is the kind of name we want to give our boys. But in the renaming, Rachel's sacrifice is lost.

Let's face it, we're all tempted to name our children Benjamin. We want to gloss over the moment when we thought of our child as Ben-Oni. We want to reserve those stories of suffering for the secret society moments when someone starts her morning sickness. But the truth is that all children are born of their mothers' suffering. It is a beautiful, Christ-like mystery. It is not to be feared or avoided. The pain of pregnancy is suffering that brings forth new life. And if we live through that life-giving pain able to tell the story, we ought to do just that.

7
Communion and Calcium Deficiency

"My body is real food."

JOHN 6:55 (NIrV)

I GREW UP IN A BAPTIST CHURCH. We didn't talk about Communion very much. If we talked about it at all, we called it the Lord's Supper. Evidently the Lord had a busy supper schedule because we only joined the Lord for supper once a quarter. Every three months the preacher would shave a few minutes off his sermon to explain that the bread and grape juice we were about to share was a symbol of Jesus' great love for us. We passed around tiny plastic cups of grape juice on shiny silver platters. We each ate a miniature square cracker. The ritual didn't seem that important. What was important was that we didn't eat this snack until we had asked the Lord Jesus into our hearts and that we, unlike the Catholics down the street, believed this meal was *only* a symbol.

Jesus said, "My flesh is real food and my blood is real drink."

The disciples responded, "This is a hard teaching. Who can accept it?" (Jn. 6:55, 60).

My church seemed to agree with the disciples.

I went to a Methodist school for seminary. We talked about Communion a lot. When we talked about it, we called it Eucharist. I learned that *Eucharist* means "thanksgiving" and that I was to be thankful for the amazing gift that Jesus gave us in his body and blood. One way to show my thanks was by coming to the Lord's Table almost every day. We would file up to the front of the chapel, hold out our hands, and receive a chunk of bread. "This is the body of Christ," the server would say. We studied how that could be true. We studied all the mental gymnastics that the church had done to explain how the bread we ate could really be Jesus' flesh. We took tests on Communion, and I learned to write fancy words like *transubstantiation*. "This is a hard teaching," I would think to myself.

Then I married a Catholic man. We talked about Communion a lot too. As a Baptist, I was not welcome at the Lord's Table in his church. We wondered if we would serve Communion at our wedding. He called it Mass, and he would cradle the wafer in his hands as if it were the most precious thing in the world. When we celebrate Communion with Protestants, he picks up the crumbs that fall from the bread, making sure to finish the bits of the meal that others leave lying around.

"It's Jesus' body," he says, as if that explains eating someone else's crumbs off an old couch. I smile warily, not knowing what to say.

"Who can accept it?" I think to myself.

When I was pregnant, I thought about eating a lot. I filled out charts about what I was eating for my midwives. I judged food according to how it would help fill my daily quotas of calcium, protein, vitamin C, and iron. I tried (with only partial success) to avoid soft cheese, and I avoided (with much more success) alcohol and caffeine. What I ate seemed important in a way it had never been before. A new life depended on what I ate.

But try as I might, I simply couldn't make myself take a multivitamin. They smelled bad, and something about swallowing a pill the size of a large insect made me throw up. My diet was nearly perfect, but I worried and worried that not taking that multivitamin was putting my child at risk of a serious birth defect. At the very least, I was sure she would be slightly less fabulous than if I had taken the multivitamin. One day, in an attempt to assuage my fears, I was researching what precisely might happen if I didn't get enough calcium each day.

I learned a startling fact—a woman's body will take calcium from her own bones to feed her baby before it allows her baby to go without the nutrients he or she needs. I was astounded. I had heard vague warnings about increased risk of osteoporosis being linked to calcium deficiency in pregnancy. I had heard an old saying that you lose a tooth for every baby you birth. But somehow I had not put it all together. My baby would eat my bones if I didn't give her enough calcium!

In one way this was reassuring. I could rest easy knowing that my child would be provided for, even if I couldn't stomach the multivitamin. In another way, the news was disconcerting. While my baby was not at risk, I was. "My body is real food," I thought.

When word got out about the Christian practice of eating Jesus' body and blood, the early church was accused of cannibalism. The accusation is understandable, but those of us who gather around the Lord's Table know that what we do is somehow different than cannibalism. Our eating does not destroy Jesus. Our eating Jesus brings us into his body, the church. Our eating Jesus gives us new life. Our eating Jesus is a way of bringing Jesus back to life among us.

The way a baby feeds off his mother is similar. At first, I felt like a little cannibal was constantly threatening to raise her fork to my bones if I didn't get in that last glass of milk each day. But I quickly realized that even with the increased risk of osteoporosis, my child's eating didn't destroy me. She could eat me, and we could both flourish. She could eat me because she lived seamlessly within my body. Her life within me revitalized my own. This sort of eating is mysterious. A baby feeds off of her mother the way we are called to feed off of Jesus. I learned to marvel at this fact soon after I gave birth to my first child.

I had been housebound for some five days and could take it no longer. I convinced my husband that a slight increase in postpartum bleeding was a small price to pay for my sanity, and we ventured out for a snail-paced walk. As we walked, we talked about how our life had changed. We neared our neighbor's house just as I admitted that I was struggling to adjust to the new constraints on my time and body.

"How *are* you?!" exclaimed my friend Amy Laura. The words poured out of her as she exploded off her front porch, arms raised to greet us and our new child. Amy Laura has a knack for drama.

"We're adjusting," I replied. "I'm lucky if I get the diapers washed and folded each day. I feel like I'm not getting anything done."

Amy Laura looked at me, aghast. Without missing a beat she trumpeted, "You have kept someone alive with your breasts! What more could you have possibly done?"

Breastfeeding is another way that mothers can offer their bodies as food, and Amy Laura rightly understands it to be important and marvelous work. Nursing was the most important thing for me to do in those days after Naomi was born. The early church also understood the importance of breastfeeding. They marveled at how a woman kept another person alive by daily offering her body as food. For medieval Christians, nursing was a powerful and common metaphor for the life of faith. Believers were understood to be like nursing babies, utterly dependent and always hungry for more spiritual nourishment. Sometimes the nursing mom in these metaphors was Mary. Sometimes the nursing mom was the spiritual leader in a community. But frequently, the mother nursing these baby Christians was Jesus himself.

Perhaps some of the reason for this easy leap from nursing moms to Jesus has to do with medieval medical theory. Medieval medicine had the science of breastfeeding a little wrong. They thought that breast milk was actually processed blood. For medieval Christians, a woman literally offered her blood to her child while nursing. Because of this understanding, it was easy for them to imagine Jesus as a breastfeeding mom.

Many of the church fathers wrote about coming to nurse at the breast of Christ. In the relationship of mother to infant, they found a profound metaphor for understanding their own relationship to Jesus. Jesus gave us his blood to drink. He promises new life to those who eat and drink of him. Moms give their blood to their babies as drink. A mother's offering sustains the life of her child on a daily basis. The connection was simple enough. In early Christian writing, images of nursing, crucifixion, and Communion are woven vividly together. Here is one example I love from a guy known as the monk of Farne. He writes:

> Little ones . . . run and throw themselves into their mothers' arms. . . . Christ our Lord does the same with us. He stretches out his hands to embrace us, bows his head down to kiss us, and opens his side to give us suck; and though it is his blood he offers us to suck we believe that it is health-giving and *sweeter than honey and the honey-comb* (Ps. 18:11). Do not wean me, good Jesus, from the *breasts of thy consolation* (Isa. 66:11). . . . It is the greatest delight to me to suck the breast of the king, who has been *my hope from the bosom of my mother, and upon whom I was cast from the womb* (Isa. 49:1, Isa. 49:23, Ps. 21:10–11). But I also need to enter again into the womb of my Lord and be reborn unto life eternal, if I am to be amongst the members of the church whose names are in the book of life.

We modern Christians tend to be so worried about a Jesus with breasts that we miss the powerful similarity between Jesus and moms. The early church didn't seem to share our gender-bending concerns. When figuring out how to communicate the gift of Christ's body, the church saw clearly that it was like the gift of a mom's body to her baby. The analogy is not limited to breastfeeding. Perhaps we can see the image of Jesus offering his body as food even more clearly in the way women feed their children while they are still in the womb.

A woman grows a whole new organ, the placenta, in order to feed her growing baby. Her blood supply increases and becomes the source of her child's food. The woman's blood flows into the placenta, bringing nutrients and oxygen to sustain her child. The woman's blood also carries away the baby's waste, so that the child can stay healthy. The woman's blood sustains life and washes away impurity. A pregnant woman's blood does for her baby what Jesus' blood does for the world. Our bones are real food, and our blood is real drink. I imagine Amy Laura exclaiming, "You kept someone alive by your blood! What more could you possibly have done?"

In John's Gospel, Jesus tries to give some explanation for *why* we must eat of his body. Jesus seems to know he is offering something a bit strange, and he takes time to explain. Jesus says:

"I am the living bread that came down from heaven. Whoever eats this bread will live forever. This bread is my flesh, which I will give for the life of the world."

Then the Jews began to argue sharply among themselves, "How can this man give us his flesh to eat?"

Jesus said to them, "Very truly I tell you, unless you eat the flesh of the Son of Man and drink his blood, you have no life in you. Whoever eats my flesh and drinks my blood has eternal life, and I will raise him up at the last day. For my flesh is real food and my blood is real drink. Whoever eats my flesh and drinks my blood remains in me, and I in them. Just as the living Father sent me and I live because of the Father, so the one who feeds on me will live because of me." (Jn. 6:51–57)

Oddly enough, I find that I understand this passage best when I substitute a pregnant woman and her child in the roles of Jesus and his followers. The example of pregnancy helps me understand something of what Jesus is asking of us. Indeed, the example of pregnancy can help to answer the question of the Jews: How can this man give us his flesh to eat? What does it take for us to be able to eat Jesus?

Jesus begins by claiming that he is living bread and that anyone who wants to live must eat of him. This is clear enough in pregnancy. A growing baby must eat of his mother in order to live. He must receive his food, nutrients, and oxygen from her blood, and he must eat them from her bones if the nutrients in the blood are not sufficient. While Jesus must insist, against our disbelief, that his flesh is *real* food and his blood is *real* drink, we can see how this is true of a mother's body and blood.

Jesus goes on to say that anyone who eats of him will be "raised up" on the last day. The Greek word used here means "to be raised up from lying down" or "to be raised from the dead." We assume Jesus means something of the latter. But the Greek word can also mean "cause to be born." We might translate Jesus' saying as, "Whoever eats my flesh and drinks my blood has eternal life, and I will cause him to be born on the last day." A mother whispers the same promise to her growing child. "Eat of me and you will live. When we come to your special day, I will cause you to be born."

Then Jesus gets to the heart of the mystery. He says, "Whoever eats my flesh and drinks my blood remains in me, and I in him." The secret of Communion is that we must live in Jesus if we want to eat of him. A baby lives inside of his mother. For the space of nine months, he "remains in her." After birth, the mother "remains in" the child. A mother smiles at her child, seeing her own features reflected, and marvels at how she "remains in him." A child is able to feed off his mother's body because they abide in one another. The indwelling of the child in the mother is what makes possible this type of intimate eating. Their mutual indwelling provides a context in which eating another becomes a life-giving joy instead of a confounding death. Mutual indwelling is a necessary part of eating Jesus.

Perhaps this is why the command to eat is so confusing. We have so few examples of people living in one another. Yet mothers and babies give us a perfect and beautiful image of how two people can "remain in one another." Jesus invites us to dwell in him the way a baby dwells in his mother. And Jesus promises to put his mark on us, to remain in us, the way a mother remains in her child after his birth. Only when we live in Jesus like a baby can we feed off of Jesus in the way he asks.

I weaned my youngest child six months ago. After three years of nonstop nursing, I was very ready for baby number two to hit the sweet potatoes and watered-down juice. (As you may have gathered, I am, at best, a faltering image of a nursing Jesus.) I assumed it would take a few weeks for my milk to dry up, but weeks came and went, and the milk kept coming. At six months postweaning, I am still producing milk.

I find this both astonishing and a bit annoying. This aging breast milk leaves crusty little nodules on my nipples that I find less than attractive. It leaks out in the shower. It leaks out when my youngest daughter claws at my shirt, yelling, "Nurse!" while I calmly explain, more for the sake of onlookers, that she doesn't nurse anymore, and I'd be happy to procure a sippy cup of virtually any liquid that does not come from my body.

For the last two months I've had a grudging relationship with this crusty old milk. I am thankful that I was able to feed my children from my body. I've marveled at how I can offer my body as food, just as Jesus offers his. But this crusty old milk seems wasted. It seems to serve no purpose at all.

I recently told my neighbor Amy Laura about my body's adamant refusal to stop producing milk. She smiled a great big smile as if it was the best news she'd heard all day.

"I'm *sure* that has religious significance," she said. I shook my head, bewildered. Her response to my souring milk seemed overly hopeful.

But I think she might be right. In the premodern world, my body's refusal to stop producing milk would have allowed me to nurse other women's children. It would have allowed me to nurse a child of one of the many women in my city who would have died in childbirth. It would have allowed me to offer my body as a gift to children besides my own. Jesus doesn't just offer his body to his biological family. Jesus throws his arms open wide. He invites all who are thirsty to come and drink.

Our culture is too squeamish and "advanced" for mothers to do much nursing of one another's babies. Formula seems a much easier option than inviting another woman into the intimacy of nursing one's child. But my milk persists as a sign of what my body is capable of offering. My crusty old milk reminds me that I'm able to give my body as food, even to children who are not my own. My milk reminds me that the gift of Jesus' body is not limited to biological family. My crusty old milk clings to me as an obnoxious sign that I am to continue giving my body for the life of the world, even after I stop nursing my own children.

"My body is real food," Jesus says.

"Mine too," I reply.

8
Expanding Bellies and the Mystery of the Church

"Abide in me, and I will abide in you."

JOHN 15:4 (ISV)

"YOUR BODY IS A TEMPLE," cautioned the well-meaning college guy who had been hired to lead our youth group through the summer. He stood before us in the requisite khaki shorts and Christian T-shirt, awkwardly trying to convince us not to have sex. Growing up in church, our youth leaders found weekly reasons to remind us that our bodies were temples. "Your body is a temple" was reason to avoid cigarettes, alcohol, sex, tattoos, and non-Christian music. We were taught that Jesus couldn't possibly live inside of us if we polluted his home. And in the Christian culture of my youth, Jesus living inside of you was the whole point of faith.

To become a Christian, I prayed a prayer inviting Jesus to come into my heart and live as the Lord of my life. As far as I could tell, there was nothing metaphorical about it. I was taught to believe that after that prayer I could say with Paul, "I no longer live, but Christ lives in me" (Gal. 2:20). I often imagined a miniature Jesus sitting right inside of me, somewhere in the middle of my chest. I imagined him pulling strings to control my movements like a master puppeteer. The fear of Jesus getting up and moving out was enough to keep me from temple polluting for most of my youth.

I understood my body to be a real home for a real Jesus. When Jesus said in John 15:4, "Abide in me, and I will abide in you," I took him at his word. But I imagined my body as something of a studio apartment. I imagined it was only big enough to house one other resident beside myself. I never imagined anyone besides Jesus moving in.

And then came Naomi.

About two weeks after I learned that Naomi was living inside of me, I found my knees on the uneven tile of our bathroom floor. It was my first bout of morning sickness, and it felt like a fire hydrant had been opened deep within me. A liquid that I'll abstain from describing was shooting out of my mouth with a force that still, even in retrospect, seems impossible.

When the rescue squad inside of me had recapped the fire hydrant, I got up, rinsed out my mouth, and knew immediately that I needed a chocolate milkshake. Specifically, I needed a chocolate milkshake made with Breyer's vanilla bean ice cream, Hershey's chocolate syrup, and skim milk. And I needed it now.

Craving isn't a strong enough word to describe the desire that was surging through my body. It was as if I had been possessed by a chocolate milkshake demon. I had the distinct sense that my body was no longer my own. As the months passed and the cravings continued, I became assured that this was indeed the case. I was no longer in charge. There was a miniature person living in me that I outweighed by at least 130 pounds, and yet, she was calling all the shots.

"I feel like a tiny tyrant has taken up residence inside of me," I explained to my husband as he made me peanut butter toast at 3 AM for the fourth night in a row.

"Maybe we should hire an exorcist," he suggested. At 3 AM the next morning, it sounded like a pretty good idea.

The uterus is a miraculous organ. Through it, women are able to welcome whole other people into their bodies to live. For nine months, women invite one, two, or even more babies to take up residence in their wombs. The same uterus can rent out space to one child and then a year later offer dual occupancy to twins. The uterus expands to make room for the size of the person living there. Not only that, the rest of the body partners with the uterus to make sure that a baby's home is as hospitable as possible. Organs scooch out of the way. Hormones work a double shift to give the body the elasticity it needs for all this movement. I think midwife Ina May Gaskin states it perfectly when she writes, "There is no other organ quite like the uterus. If men had such an organ, they would brag about it. So should we."

My uterus allowed me to become a literal home for another person. In pregnancy, my body was more clearly a temple than it had ever been before. Naomi's presence in me was even more motivational for life change than Jesus' presence had been. I quickly changed my diet and daily habits to create a welcoming space for her to live. The youth leaders had warned that cigarettes and alcohol were temple pollutants, and while I'd never been able to figure out why Jesus would care about those, it was clear that Naomi needed a temple free of such toxins. When Naomi said rest, I rested. I even gave up soft cheese, something God knows I would never do for him.

I learned more deeply than I'd ever known before that my body was indeed residential space. I became a home. My body was a temple.

But Jesus doesn't just ask to live in us. Allowing Jesus to live in us is only half the mystery. The other half is that Jesus asks us to live in him. "Abide in me, and I will abide in you," he says. We know how to welcome Jesus into our bodies because Jesus first welcomed us into his.

While I was primarily taught as a young Baptist that being a Christian meant letting Jesus live in me, my husband was primarily taught as a young Catholic the other half of the mystery: that being a Christian meant dwelling in Christ's body, the church. For him, the church is the body of Jesus, plain and simple. Each of us is invited in.

We don't have lots of examples of people living inside one another. Pregnancy is perhaps the best example we have of one person welcoming another into her body the way Jesus asks us to live in him. Like a uterus, Christ's body expands to make room for whoever comes. The early church understood this connection and explicitly imagined Jesus having a womb. One tradition even depicts Mary living in the womb of Jesus, her son. In a poem about this image, St. Ephrem writes, "O Christ, you have given birth to your own mother in the second birth that comes from water."

Coptic Christians understand that the church is the body of Christ so deeply that they shape their church buildings to look like Jesus' body. The church is formed in the shape of a cross, with the altar being Christ's head and the end of the cross being Christ's feet. The congregation enters from the side. They understand themselves to be entering through the wound in Christ's side. The place where the congregation sits is understood to be Christ's womb. They believe that Christ's *wound* opened a way for them to enter Christ's *womb* for worship.

So let's admit it, Jesus having a womb sounds a little creepy. We want to join Nicodemus in mocking Jesus' suggestion that we be born again. We want to join Nicodemus in his sarcasm as he asks Jesus, "Would you have us enter our mother's womb a second time?" As far as we're concerned, living in a womb is a once-in-a-lifetime event that we have no interest in redoing.

But Jesus says, "Abide in me." And the early church understood that when Jesus welcomes us into himself, he looks like a pregnant woman. And if Jesus looks like a pregnant woman, we Christians are called to look something like twins.

While I was pregnant with my second child, three of the guys from my youth group began their families. At roughly the same time, all of their wives got pregnant with twins. There were lots of jokes about something in the water. Knowing how much water I'd shared with these guys made me more than slightly worried. I had always thought of twins as a rare phenomenon, but my odds at getting a set of my own seemed to be rising all too quickly.

I got a few e-mail updates about their pregnancies. Ultrasound pictures were sent of two tiny people touching hands, resting in each other's arms, and snuggling with each other in the small home they shared. One day I opened my inbox to a very short e-mail from one of the couples, John and Liz. At twenty-eight weeks gestation, their twins had died. John wrote, "We are taking comfort in the fact that neither of our children died alone. They lived their lives playing together. They died in each others arms."

Christians are called to live in Jesus the way these little twins lived in Liz. We are called to live together so closely and intimately that we share everything in common. Acts 2:44 describes the early Christians by saying, "All the believers were together and had everything in common." Acts describes a group of people who met together each day to eat and pray. They opened their homes to one another. They sold their possessions to provide for each other's needs. The early church lived scrunched up in the womb of Christ, glad to be so close together. When they died, they died in each others arms.

While it's hard for us to imagine Jesus with a womb, it seems just as hard for us to imagine ourselves as twins. We simply aren't willing to share our lives with others that intimately. We're afraid that we won't get a fair share of the food. We're afraid it will be too cramped if we live with other people in one house. So we build our own houses instead of moving into the womb of Christ. We buy our own food instead of living off Jesus' placenta. We keep our distance instead of living scrunched up with other Christians. And we miss out on what it means to be the church.

Jesus was clear that the kingdom of God belongs to little children. In Mark 10:15 Jesus says, "Truly I tell you, anyone who will not receive the kingdom of God like a little child will never enter it."

Sharing is a difficult lesson to learn. Sometimes, I'm tempted to think that my girls (and most toddlers I know) are very poor sharers. When I most want them to share, they are prone to fling their bodies on the ground, writhing in fits of agony, as if taking turns with a sticky plastic doll is the greatest injustice I could have ever concocted. These fits tempt me to think that Jesus didn't know what he was talking about. Should we enter the kingdom with grabbing, biting, hair-pulling fits?

But in other ways, when they don't know I'm looking, my girls share life so intimately that it makes me squeamish. Fay will gnaw on an animal cracker until it's a fistful of mush, and then offer it to Naomi. Naomi's eyes light up as she exclaims, "Thank you!" and crams the mush in her mouth. They resist my unending attempts to make them say "sorry," but they have developed their own ritual for asking forgiveness. In it, they lick each other's cheeks while the offender rubs the victim's tummy, saying, "Wiggle, wiggle!" While the ritual is far, far beyond my comprehension, there is a warmth and vulnerability to it that no forced "sorry" has ever achieved. One Friday night, in an attempt at a bit of alone time, my husband and I put the girls in front of a movie. We came to check on them a bit later to find the girls sharing a chair. Fay was asleep in her sister's arms.

Children, like twins in utero and like the early Christians in Acts, know how to share their food, space, and life with an intimacy that makes us cringe. Jesus calls it the church. He calls their sharing blessed. He throws open his side and invites us to crawl in and live cramped up together inside of him. And then, while we're still reeling from the invitation to all this cramped and sticky sharing, Jesus asks us to go and do likewise. Jesus asks us to invite in others as he has invited in us.

My Baptist faith asked me to welcome Jesus, but it didn't stress that Jesus might want me to welcome others as well. We recited John 3:16 like our lives depended on it, but we didn't read Matthew 25 very often. In it, Jesus explains that welcoming the least among us is just like welcoming him. Jesus explains that he expects us to welcome others the way we would welcome him. Jesus explains that welcoming others is at the very heart of what it means to be a Christian. Salvation depends upon our willingness to welcome others as Christ.

Matthew 25:31–46 tells a story in which Jesus separates the blessed and the cursed. But no one in the story can figure out how they got to be on the blessed or cursed side of things. So Jesus takes time to explain. He says to the blessed, "Come . . . take your inheritance. . . . For I was hungry and you gave me something to eat, I was thirsty, and you gave me something to drink, I was a stranger and you invited me in, I needed clothes and you clothed me, I was sick and you looked after me, I was in prison and you came to visit me."

The blessed can't figure out when they did all of this for Jesus. Jesus replies, "Truly I tell you, whatever you did for one of the least of these brothers and sisters of mine, you did for me."

Matthew 25 is like a mission statement for the church. It includes explicit instructions for what we are to be about in the world. When I take time to read it, I am inspired to volunteer at the soup kitchen, to let folks without homes stay at my house, and to get rid of much of my excess clothing that others might at least have enough.

Rarely do I feel motivated to take care of my own kids after reading Matthew 25. But the truth is, our relationships with our own children can be the best training ground for the practices of feeding, clothing, and welcoming.

One day we read this passage in Bible study with our friends Jackie and Jeremy. Jackie and Jeremy have four boys under the age of six. As we read the familiar words of Matthew 25, Jeremy interrupted.

"I do all of this with my kids," he said. "They're naked, sick, hungry, and if not quite strangers, they're definitely strange." Jeremy went on to explain that doing these acts of care for strangers was sometimes easier than doing them day after day in his own home. But doing these acts in our own home is as much at the heart of Christian faith as doing them at the soup kitchen. If we can do them in our own home, then we can learn to do them outside of our home with the genuine love and respect we offer our children. We can learn to feed, clothe, and welcome with an intimacy we rarely take to service projects.

Pregnant women perform these acts of welcoming in their own bodies. Our babies are strangers to us and we invite them inside of us to live. They are in need of food and we give it. They come out naked and we have a well-chosen Onesie waiting. And yet we understand our babies as a breathtaking gift, as immeasurably worthy. When we kiss their faces for the first time, it is easy to feel like we are kissing the face of God.

The challenge is to extend our acts of feeding, clothing, and welcoming beyond our own children. The challenge is to believe that each hungry person, not just our own little one, is Christ. The challenge is to welcome those without homes with the same intimacy and vulnerability we use in welcoming our children into our very bodies. The challenge is to select clothes for those in need with the care we use in selecting the clothes we give our children.

The mystery at the heart of the church is that we are called to let Jesus abide in us. The scandal at the heart of the church is that Jesus doesn't come alone. He comes dragging a whole bunch of other folks with him. He asks us to let him and his crew live in us, and he asks us to come live in him, cramped up with the same higgledy-piggledy crew.

"Abide in me, and I will abide in you," Jesus says.

It sounds crazy. But we pregnant women and our babies do it every day.

PART THREE
Birthing the Fruit of the Spirit

9
Learning the Logic of the Kingdom

---

*"So the last will be first, and the
first will be last."*

MATTHEW 20:16

"YOU'LL BOUNCE BACK," SAID THE MIDDLE-AGED, obnoxiously optimistic woman who had just asked me how I was feeling. At eighteen months after the birth of back-to-back baby number two, I don't bounce anywhere. I sort of sluggishly drag myself from place to place. Maybe the gooey stick of whatever my girls last ate and smeared on me is clogging my gears. Or maybe three years of sleep deprivation is turning me into a zombie. No one ever expects a zombie to bounce. Or maybe the idea that anyone can "bounce back" from pregnancy is just untrue and unhelpful at its core.

My youngest child is eighteen months old, and my body is still recovering. I still have back pain that doctors attribute to back-to-back pregnancies. I still get headaches attributed to hormonal shifts. And I have recently added an autoimmune response to my IUD triggered by weaning to the list of afflictions. In lay terms, that has meant that every month since I weaned Fay I get random inflammation in different parts of my body and a sore throat the week before my period. Bouncing is not in my foreseeable future.

But as much as I hate the phrase, I think I might have experienced something of what people mean by it after my first child's birth. Around six months after Naomi was born, I woke up one morning feeling strong. My midsection felt empty, even sort of flat. I got out of bed without rolling over and using the gravity of my legs to pull the rest of me up. I actually just sat up, using my core muscles without any sort of pain, resistance, or that odd bulge in the center of the stomach that doctors warn you'll see if you try to do crunches too early. I stood up, and my back seemed able to carry my weight easily. It was a miracle, and not a minor one.

"I feel like myself again!" I announced as I walked triumphantly into the kitchen.

That morning inaugurated a blessed two months of using upbeat exercise videos without peeing myself. I started praying in the mornings, still had energy for small tasks at night, and even found myself wanting to have sex more than once a month. I also remember distinctly thinking, "It wouldn't be so horrible if I got pregnant again." In the previous six months, the thought of getting pregnant again literally made me nauseous. I could easily start a snot-producing, heaving sob just thinking about the possibility. But the morning I woke up feeling light and strong and able, I could imagine going through the whole ordeal of pregnancy again. And it felt good.

We knew we wanted to have a second child sometime in the coming years. We knew we didn't want to deal with hormone-based birth control for such a short period of time. So I had gotten a diaphragm, and Dan had a box of condoms, and before the day I woke up feeling like Martha Stewart on steroids, we honestly just didn't have much sex. But as I got back a bit of the bounce in my step and started imagining having another child, we became a bit lax in our use of the diaphragm. The condoms just never seemed to be quite where we needed them to be. I kept loose track of my cycle, and we tried halfheartedly not to have sex when I was fertile. But after two months of feeling myself again, I found myself pregnant with baby number two. My bounce left with the first bout of morning sickness.

Naomi was eight months old when I got pregnant with Fay. I had planned to nurse Naomi for at least a year, if not longer, so I called our birthing center to find out if they had any advice about breastfeeding while pregnant. The nurse offered me the usual advice: plenty of fluids, good diet, daily multivitamin. But then she gave me a word of "encouragement." She said, "You don't have to worry about your body knowing what to do. Whenever you eat, your body will feed the growing baby first, your current baby second, and you last."

I sighed with relief. The nurse was trying to assuage my fear that nursing my eight-month-old would take nutrients from the new baby I had just learned was growing inside of me. It worked. I felt better. Or rather, I felt better for approximately seven seconds. Then I realized that this put me last on the food chain.

I could feel a mild panic building at the edge of my temples. I imagined fat little babies pushing their emaciated mother away from the dinner table as they gobbled everything in sight. And then I heard a calm, clear voice say, "The first will be last." The waves of panic began to ebb away.

I had heard this phrase repeated in church my whole life. I had heard it said jokingly by the folks in the back of the line at church supper. I had heard it interchanged with a phrase like it: the least shall be greatest. I had heard it preached as something of a mandate, a fundamental rule to guide Christian living. I had heard Sunday school teachers skillfully talk around the phrase until it was robbed of its scandal and power.

"The first will be last."

Jesus says this in Matthew's Gospel as he is teaching his disciples what his kingdom will be like. Jesus means it as good news. But rarely is it received as such. No one wants to be last. At my best, I take this verse to mean that everyone is equal in God's sight. But I have a sneaking suspicion that Jesus is up to something far more odd than that. Read straightforwardly, Jesus says that in his kingdom the whole order of things will be turned upside down. The least among us will be valued as the greatest. Those who are weak will have their needs met first. Those who are first will be last in line. Those who work for one hour will be paid the same as those who work all day. Everyone will go home with a paycheck that can support their family.

The disciples don't like this saying any more than I do. Jesus has to repeat it twice (Matt. 19:30; 20:16). We struggle to take Jesus seriously on this point. We don't know how to give up our privilege, especially when we feel we have earned it by hard work. Yet pregnant bodies have this godly logic written into their very DNA.

Even without a woman's consent, a pregnant body sees the weakness and dependence of a developing fetus and decides that such a little one should be fed first. Then the body sees a drooly, just-crawling eight-month-old and, without a second thought, feeds that child next. Then the body passes the leftovers to the woman who put the fork to her mouth in the first place. And usually, there is enough for all. But if someone has to do without, the mother is the one best prepared to make that nutritional sacrifice. We struggle to put Jesus' logic to work in our lives, but pregnant, breastfeeding mothers do it every time they eat. These mothers model how it can be good news that the least among us are fed first.

The most remarkable thing about this sacrifice is that our bodies do it for us. My body makes a decision that I'm not sure I would otherwise make. Now I'm sure there are some moms out there who would have stopped at relief when the nurse delivered this nutritional fun-fact. I'm sure there are moms who would be serenely overjoyed to know that their bodies will naturally feed two people ahead of them every time they lift a fork to their lips. But I'm not that mom. I have enough selfishness left in me to know that I do not want to be last in the church potluck line eating the cold dregs of green bean casserole with no crunchies left on top. And I definitely don't want to do that every time I sit down to eat. But my body puts me last in line anyway. I have no choice in the matter.

When I was in youth group, we sang a song (over and over and over again) that said, "My spirit is willing, but my flesh is so weak." We were warned to stay away from fleshly temptations. We read from Romans 8:5–6 (NRSV), "For those who live according to the flesh set their minds on the things of the flesh, but those who live according to the Spirit set their minds on the things of the Spirit. To set the mind on the flesh is death, but to set the mind on the Spirit is life and peace." And we read on to find that "if you live according to the flesh, you will die; but if by the Spirit you put to death the deeds of the body, you will live" (Rom. 8:13). Somewhere in all that reading and singing, I got the clear impression that my body was a problem. It was the source of sin, and if I had my head on straight, I wouldn't trust it.

I'm sure there is some truth to this. Let's admit it, some of us are pregnant because there is some truth to this. But somewhere along the way, our churches got so good at warning against the weakness of the flesh, that we've overlooked how our bodies can be a means of grace. If my spirit had anything to do with it, I would *not* be last on the food chain. But my body knows that my spirit is weak, and so she didn't check in for permission. Instead, my body went ahead and followed God's command. Pregnant bodies innately know and practice the ways of God. Pregnant bodies follow the logic of God's kingdom. Pregnant flesh isn't as weak as we are tempted to think it is.

So why aren't our churches holding up pregnant women as models for the life of faith? To the church's credit, the role of mothers in Scripture is confusing. There are a few places in the Bible where Jesus even seems to disparage his own mother or mothers generally. No wonder the church has had difficulty making sense of the role of moms in the kingdom of God.

But when we look more closely at these stories that seem disparaging, there is something deeper at work. I think Jesus is offering us moms a little advice about what to do with this wisdom our bodies are teaching us.

In Luke 11:27–28 Jesus has just healed a demon-possessed man and is teaching about the significance of what he has done. A woman yells out from the crowd, "Blessed is the mother who gave you birth and nursed you!" Jesus replies, "Blessed rather are those who hear the word of God and obey it."

Here is a woman, probably a mother herself, who is so overwhelmed by Jesus' teaching that she makes a public affirmation of how glad she is to have Jesus around. Her exclamation, as I take it, means something like, "I'm so glad you are in the world! Blessed is the woman who made it possible for you to be here!" But instead of receiving her comment politely, as all mothers hope their children would do, Jesus turns the comment on its head. He takes the comment as a teaching moment. But in doing so, he seems to slight the role of mothers and make light of this woman's blessing.

It's almost as bad as when Jesus publicly insults his mother in Matthew 12:46–50. Jesus is out teaching again, and Mary and his brothers are waiting to speak with him. Someone informs him that his family is waiting, and Jesus responds, "Who is my mother, and who are my brothers?" Pointing to his disciples, he says, "Here are my mother and my brothers. For whoever does the will of my Father in heaven is my brother and sister and mother."

Really, Jesus? Everyone who does the will of your Father bore sciatic nerve pain to bring you into the world? Everyone who does the will of your Father labored in a barn on scratchy hay to hear your first cries? Everyone who does the will of your Father faithfully nursed a colicky baby messiah?

What is Jesus up to? Not only is he not telling the world about how mothers are model disciples, he even seems to put mothers down. This is not what we mothers would hope for from the Son of God! But Jesus is doing some important theological work, albeit in a somewhat rude fashion. In both of these passages, Jesus is insisting that there is nothing exclusive about the family of God. Anyone who hears the word of God and obeys it can be blessed. Anyone who does the will of God can be in Jesus' family. Jesus knows his followers well. He knows that we are quick to show special favor to our own. We are quick to give our blessings to our biological families. But the blessings of Jesus' kingdom know no biological boundaries.

Pregnant bodies know the logic of the kingdom. Without ever asking us to make a choice, our bodies make the least greatest and the first last. But our bodies only do that for our own babies. It is a beautiful, holy, profound act, but it has its limits. If we only extend the logic of the kingdom to our own children, we really aren't living into the abundance of God's vision. We must let our bodies teach us how to treat not only our own babies, but the whole world around us.

In pregnancy, we learn sacrificial love for our own babies. Jesus says, "The kid next door is your baby too." Then Jesus insists that the child in the neighborhood we don't even drive through is also our baby. Then he insists that the child who makes fun of our own child on the playground is also our baby! We are to extend the logic that our bodies taught us in pregnancy to that obnoxious little brat as well. And once we learn all that, perhaps we can learn to put the first last in other arenas of life. After all, Jesus was originally talking about economics when he introduced this particularly difficult saying.

Jesus doesn't have anything against moms. But Jesus wants to make sure that we mothers extend the lessons our bodies learn in pregnancy beyond our own biological children.

This section of the book is titled "Birthing the Fruit of the Spirit." The fruits of the spirit are those things we need to live the life of faith well. Sometimes we call them the armor of God. Sometimes we call them spiritual disciplines. When I say "fruit of the Spirit," I mean to include any practice, attitude, or spiritual gift that helps us hold on to God in the messiness of our daily lives. In other words, this section of the book is about how pregnancy teaches us those disciplines. Pregnancy teaches us a new way to worship. It teaches us how to wait. Pregnancy teaches us to believe in the unseen and to live by grace. Pregnancy teaches us how to live into the truth that the least will be greatest and the first will be last. Pregnancy teaches us that these audacious claims of Jesus are possible in the real world. Our task is to take these lessons that our bodies know innately and apply them to life after pregnancy. If we let our faithfulness stop at our own families, we miss the radical invitation to enter the family of God.

We have a potluck dinner at our house every Tuesday night. All sorts of people come: friends, neighborhood kids, folks that need free food. Not everyone brings a dish, but we call it a potluck in the hopes that some will. We get some ten to twenty-five guests on any given week. I must admit that I am rarely the last in line. I am sometimes the first in line, and a few of those times, I'm not even making one of my children's plates! I am instead, even though I'm sure it's wrong, trying to get the crunchy part of the green bean casserole or the fresh garden tomatoes perched atop the salad. I am a grudging disciple at best.

But even when I'm taking more than my share of the garden tomatoes, Tuesday nights are my attempt to let the fetus eat first. Tuesday nights are when I let other people sit on my couch and use my dishes and trample the white rug in my bathroom. I realize white is a bad choice for a bathmat. I made that color choice with full knowledge that I would have to wash the silly thing all too frequently. But it still irks me to no end when people put their dirt on my pearly white bathmat. But even though I know that whoever comes will dirty my bath mat, I spend the afternoon cooking for them anyway. I pray as I cook, asking that each who comes will be fed in whatever way they need feeding. I extend my mothering to folks outside my biological family. I try to do what my body did so well in feeding Fay first, Naomi second, and myself last. I shove my own desires for a clean house aside and open my table to the family of God. Each Tuesday night, the family of God is gracious enough to accept the invitation. And when they do, my spirit slowly learns what my body knows already—the upside-down logic of the kingdom of God.

10
The Mystery of Faith

—

*"Now faith is being sure of what we hope for
and certain of what we do not see."*

HEBREWS 11:1 (NIV 1984)

*"My grace is sufficient for you, for my power
is made perfect in weakness."*

2 CORINTHIANS 12:9

MY FRIENDS SCOTT AND SHEILA ARE A SUPER-COOL
husband-and-wife photography team. They buy their clothes
at thrift stores and look like they are about to take the stage
at an indie rock concert. When I shop at thrift stores, I end up
looking like a sixty-year-old high school science teacher. Sheila
sews intriguing accents onto everything in their home and
paints gorgeous banners and posters for nearly every event.
They have an eye for beauty. So of course we were ecstatic
when they offered to take the photographs for our wedding.

"It will be our gift," said Sheila. Her bright eyes laughed as
she graciously shrugged off my attempts to offer payment.

Sheila had been pregnant for about four months when our
wedding day came around. I hadn't seen her since early in

her pregnancy. When we had last met, she was seriously struggling with morning sickness. She had joked that she might never gain any weight if her food continued to evacuate her body immediately after consumption. I worried that she might be right. The last time I saw her she was still as skinny as Barbie's kid sister.

Two hours before the wedding, I came outside in my flouncy white dress to see Sheila clicking away on her camera in the excruciating North Carolina summer heat. I watched her from behind as she took pictures of my mother directing the placement of flower arrangements. I thought to myself that she looked as skinny as ever. And then she turned around.

It looked as if a basketball had been fastened right to the front of her tummy. Not a full-size basketball, mind you. More like a pool-size basketball. A perfectly round bump protruding off her tiny frame. I laughed out loud. She ran over to me, and I grabbed the tiny ball of a belly. In my wedding day glee, I let my awe at how her body was changing run free. To top it all off, I exclaimed, "Oh my gosh, you're really pregnant!"

"I know!" laughed Sheila. "I was just starting to think it was all a mistake and that I had a really serious case of food poisoning when this little ball popped out. I guess we really are having a baby!"

A short five months later, I would find myself exclaiming something of the same.

We conceived Naomi just a month and a half after our wedding day. My nausea started as early as nausea can possibly start. But right around week fourteen the nausea let up and I found myself in an odd sort of calm. I knew I was pregnant, but I had no daily signs that it was truly the case. My pants were tighter, but they still fit. When I looked in the mirror, I didn't look pregnant per se. I had the unpleasant suspicion that I looked like someone who had been stress eating disproportionate amounts of Ben and Jerry's ice cream. My first trimester had been like a raging storm of hormones and vomit. But now the seas of my body were calm. After about a week of this quiet, I started to wonder if I hadn't made the whole thing up.

"Are we sure I'm pregnant?" I asked my husband.

"We're sure," he answered, barely looking up from his book to acknowledge my confusion about the lack of symptoms.

I fought the urge to take more pregnancy tests. I pined for the next doctor's appointment when I would hear the baby's heartbeat. I felt around in my abdomen each morning for the hard ball my mom had said would eventually rise up toward my ribs. I lay perfectly still on the couch after dinner waiting to feel the first fluttery kick. But nothing came.

My pregnancy books said that most women would feel their babies kick sometime between sixteen and twenty weeks. I had heard that skinny women sometimes feel their babies even earlier.

"Do I qualify as skinny?" I asked my husband.

My prenatal yoga teacher (who definitely qualifies as skinny) had described how she was so in tune with her body that she actually felt her baby kick around week fourteen. I spent weeks fourteen and fifteen meditating on my uterus. I sat in lotus pose and invited my child to give me a sign of his or her existence. Nothing happened. I lay on my back with my hips in the air and meditated on my uterus. Nothing happened. I stood in mountain pose, grounding my feet into the worn-out carpet and breathed deeply into my uterus. Still, nothing.

"Would you say I'm more or less in tune with my body than the average woman?" I asked my husband.

By week twenty-one I still had no visible sign that I was pregnant. I was outside the outer range for feeling my baby kick, and I still felt nothing. I had decided I was neither skinny nor in tune with my body, but I had been to the doctor and heard my child's heart beating wildly. Sign or no sign, I was pregnant.

"Now faith is being sure of what we hope for and certain of what we do not see." I memorized this verse as a child. I learned to say it in a rhythmic, sing-song voice that we used to say all of our weekly verses in Sunday school. I had learned to say the reference, Hebrews 11:1, in the same sing-song rhythm after reciting the verse. But all of the reciting hadn't made the substance of the verse any easier to accept.

I like evidence. I have little patience for promises. I say to my husband, "I'll believe it when I see it," more often than he likes. As far as I'm concerned, the unseen might as well not exist. I'll be quite happy to engage the unseen when it reveals itself to the naked eye, thank you very much.

But the Bible has no space for my results-based, believe-it-when-I-see-it realism. To my dogged desire for proof, the Bible repeats, "Now faith is being sure of what we hope for and certain of what we do not see." Pregnancy echoes this scriptural refrain.

At some point during pregnancy, most women struggle with feeling unpregnant. For some women it happens in the first days of pregnancy when our babies seem to be nothing more than a light pink line on a pee stick. For those women who manage to escape nausea, it happens in the first few months. For me, it happened after my nausea subsided but before I could feel my baby moving within me. We struggle with the oddity that something huge is happening within us while we have no immediate proof that the something huge really exists. We wonder at why we've changed our lives, our diets, and our daily habits on behalf of a little person we can't even see. We buy an arsenal of stuff to create a comfortable space for a little child who refuses to give us even one fluttery kick. We learn to be sure of what we hope for and certain of what we do not see. In short, pregnant women have faith.

Faith is a funny word. It is one of the words I have come to call "church words." Church words are those words that get thrown around church like candy on Halloween. We can't seem to get through a sentence without using one. When I was growing up in youth group, a few of the guys would raise their hands to answer questions before they were even asked. They'd shout with exceptional speed, "God, love, Jesus!" They had learned that whatever the question, one of those words was probably the answer. Those are church words.

Grace . . . salvation . . . righteousness . . . belief . . . faith. We say these words so much that we never bother to stop and define them. We assume we know what they mean, but when pressed for a definition, I have found that church words occupy a pretty fuzzy spot in my brain. "Now faith is being sure of what we hope for . . . " I'm not sure that I actually know what that means.

For most of my life, I was afraid to let anyone know that most of these church words didn't seem entirely clear. I worried that if I told my pastor that I didn't know what *faith* meant, he would promptly inform me that I must not have any. But then I took a class with a quirky New Testament professor from New Zealand. Dr. Campbell knows more about the apostle Paul than anyone I've ever met. He talks about Paul as if they'd been fishing together just last week. I got the impression that if I asked him the color of the tunic Paul was wearing when he wrote the letter to the Romans, Dr. Campbell might actually know. So I was relieved to hear Dr. Campbell say that he didn't like the word *faith* either. Paul uses the word some 140 times in the Bible, but Dr. Campbell didn't think "faith" was a good translation for the Greek word that Paul actually used.

"I'm not entirely sure what 'faith' really means," he said. "I think a better translation would be something like 'trust.'"

The day I heard these words from Dr. Campbell, I started a little experiment. Whenever I saw the word *faith* in my Bible, I substituted the word *trust* in my mind. And it was as if I had a whole new Bible. For me, trust requires a lot more of me than faith. Trust is Aladdin reaching out his hand to Princess Jasmine, asking her to jump off a ten-story palace, and saying, "Do you trust me?" Trust is my parents saying, "We trust you," when they handed me the keys to the car and let my little sister get in for the first time. Trust is what I do when I let my husband fix the plumbing even though I know the whole house could end up under a foot of water. "I trust you," I say as I put our home into his hands.

In my experience, *faith* is a heady word, a spiritual word, some sort of internal state. But trust involves risk. Trust means giving over your stuff, your loved ones, even your own body to the care of another. Trust means depending on others when it seems easier and safer to depend on yourself. Faith might start as belief in the unseen, but the fullness of faith is trusting that unseen God to provide for your needs in very tangible, visible ways.

Pregnancy teaches the trusting sort of faith, too.

"One, two, three, four . . . " the nurse counted to ten slowly and calmly while my sister pushed through the contraction. I was holding her foot in my hand with her calf cradled in my forearm. Her impeccably polished toenails looked slick in the fluorescent hospital light. When Lisa was little, our grandfather called her "puff ball." With her puff of wispy blond curls and her slight frame, we joked that she could be blown away by the wind. But her leg seemed heavy now. I was holding the leg of a full-grown woman, and the little blond puff was nowhere to be found.

My mother held Lisa's other leg, and her husband Rob supported her from behind. Lisa had hoped to give birth without medication, and she had labored beautifully for some twenty-five hours without any pain relief. But for some reason, her cervix actually seemed to be closing, and we had run out of ideas for how to help labor progress.

"She needs an epidural to relax her cervix and enable labor to continue," the nurse had said matter-of-factly.

We looked at each other, wondering if this was true. I could see the frustration in my mother's face that we didn't know more about the mechanics of labor. I pushed down my frustration at not having the knowledge to help my sister. Lisa sighed and did what she had become accustomed to doing. She made the best decision for her child with the information available to her. My mother and I were directed to wait outside until the epidural was in place.

Some four hours and a Pitocin drip later, Lisa was fully dilated and ready to push. But because of the epidural she couldn't feel her contractions or lift her own legs. The nurse positioned Rob, mom, and me to help. We're not normally a touchy family, but Lisa smiled at each of us as we took hold of her body. She joked that we were doing as much work as she was. The unplanned epidural had left her immobile, but she graciously accepted our help as we maneuvered her body into a good position for pushing.

After a few pushes, Ezra's head was visible. And by head, I really mean hair. A thick, black mass of hair was inching its way forward. As his head would dip back inside her body, a little strand of hair was left hanging outside of my sister. We laughed and joked and held up a mirror for Lisa to see the tiny wig her baby was sporting in utero. We told her how well she was doing and reminded each other to push her legs back against her chest. The nurse massaged her perineum with each push, and my mom reminded Lisa to keep her chin to her chest. Just as we were settling into a straightforward and surprisingly joyous second-stage labor, the nurse announced that she was going to leave to find the doctor. My mother and I looked at each other, a bit confused.

"Should we keep pushing without you?" my mom asked.

"Sure," the nurse said brightly. She seemed unconcerned at leaving Ezra's increasingly visible wig in our care.

"Great!" said Mom, trying to mirror the nurse's confidence.

Mom was trained as a nurse and had given birth to three children. I had given birth to both my girls within the last three years and had recently supported one of my friends during her labor. Mom had been with me for the birth of both of my girls. Surely we could babysit these emerging black curls for a few moments in the nurse's absence.

As the nurse disappeared, I took her place between my sister's legs. Rob took hold of my previously assigned leg and adjusted the bed to support Lisa's back. By the next contraction, we were in our new positions. I counted calmly and slowly to ten, just as I'd heard the nurse do. Mom and Rob pushed back on Lisa's legs, and Lisa bore down hard, settling into her newfound strength. The little black wig came swirling out.

"Um, he's not leaving," I said. Worry and excitement flooded my body. I looked at my mom, who seemed to be battling the same mix of emotions.

"Should I be giving perineal support?" I asked, hoping my mom's age meant she would know what to do.

Mom nodded vigorously. I grabbed a towel and pressed against Lisa, right below the little black wig. I counted again, fighting to keep my voice calm, and the little black wig inched out more. The wet ringlets brushed against my hand, and tears sprung to my eyes. Just when I thought my little nephew might fall into my hands, the nurse came back into the room.

"Whoa!" she exclaimed, rushing in front of me. "This is *not* how I left you all!"

"You told us to keep pushing!" my mother and I protested simultaneously.

Neither of us responds well to being treated like disobedient second graders, but just as we were gearing up to defend our successful communal effort at bringing Ezra into the world, a flurry of nurses filled the room. I grabbed the video and film cameras. Previous to delivering Ezra or holding Lisa's right leg, I had been tasked with recording the birth. I filmed in one hand and snapped pictures in the other so that Lisa could look back and remember the work she had done.

The story of Ezra's birth is the story of Lisa's accomplishment. But it's also the story of Lisa's willingness to depend upon others for help. Her story of strength is also a story of being held up by her husband, mother, sister, and a host of nurses. The story of Ezra's birth is the story of Lisa's faith.

Pregnant women learn throughout pregnancy to trust others for their basic needs. They learn their own limits. They learn to ask for and receive help. They learn to surround themselves with communities of support, knowing that when they most need to, they might not be able to lift their own legs. They learn to trust that God will meet their needs through the people around them. In short, pregnant women learn to live by faith.

Living by faith isn't easy. Most of us don't want to ask for help. We don't want to be dependent. It feels very vulnerable to let others (even our partners!) see our weakness. We don't know if they'll honor that weakness or exploit it—if they'll help us in our need or dismiss us as high-maintenance nuisances. It is risky business to believe that God's grace is sufficient to meet our needs, that God's power is made perfect in weakness (2 Cor. 12:9).

We like to think that being Christian is about helping other people. It feels good to meet the needs of others. But being a Christian is equally about learning to let others help us. Jesus asks his disciples to leave their jobs and families to follow him, not knowing where their next meal will come from. God asks Abraham to leave family and homeland on the absurd promise that in his old age he will have a child who will become a great nation. The Israelites leave slavery in Egypt only to wander around in a desert, depending on God to provide every single meal. The Bible is full of stories of God asking folks to leave their self-built support systems to live lives of dependence in which God meets their basic daily needs. This sort of seemingly foolish, extremely uncomfortable willingness to lean upon God is at the heart of Christian faith. Our willingness to be weak, vulnerable, and dependent is truly the space in which God's power is seen.

Our bodies know that we don't want to appear weak or vulnerable. Our bodies also know that we will need to depend on other people during our labors. As labor intensifies, our bodies naturally decrease our inhibitions. Thus, a woman who might usually insist on wearing a T-shirt over her bathing suit can labor completely naked with no less than three people in the room, most of whom are touching her at any given time.

My husband's favorite memory of my labor with Naomi reflects this natural lessening of inhibitions. In birthing class we had been taught that contractions begin slowly and gradually increase over a period of hours. Naomi's labor was nothing like the textbook labor we had been taught. Instead, labor slammed in hard and fast with contractions lasting a full minute with barely space to breathe in between. Our childbirth educator, Cherri, had suggested that we use the space in between contractions to gather our belongings and make our way to the car.

"Don't leave mom during a contraction," she had cautioned the birth partners. "Take the four to six minutes that you have between contractions to get things ready."

"Don't try to walk to the car during a contraction," she had cautioned the moms. "Wait until a contraction is over, then leave immediately and try to be settled in the car for the next contraction."

We had no such luxury. With only a ninety-second break, Dan couldn't help but be away during my contractions. Of course, in my laboring state, I took his absence as flagrant refusal to follow our birth plan. After realizing that screaming for him only increased my pain, I threw at the door everything I could reach from my location on the bathroom floor to get his attention and indicate my displeasure at his absence.

But when I attempted to make my way to the car, I found out what a bind he had been in. In the space between two contractions, Dan told me that the car was ready. I waited for the contraction to end. As soon as it did, I stood up quickly and started walking to the door. Dan gently informed me that I had on neither underwear nor shoes. I waved him off, annoyed that he would bring attention to so small a matter at a time like this. It was after midnight, and somewhere in the back of my mind I assured myself that no one would see me. In Dan's nonlaboring mind, he was aware of the fact that we live in a highly populated neighborhood on a street corner that hosts a fairly active nightlife.

I made it to the sidewalk when another contraction seized the middle of my body. I dropped to the concrete on all fours. In telling the story, my husband is quick to point out that I was directly under a street lamp, and my bare bottom was shining for all to see. I'm not convinced that is such an important detail to share, but since I'm telling his favorite memory, I feel I should keep it in. When the contraction ended, I made my way into the car. Routine inhibition was nowhere to be found.

I ripped off my shirt as soon as we got to the birth center, thankful to be in a place where no unnecessary nuisances like shirts were required. For nine hours, I paced the room without a stitch of clothing on. Dan and my mother held my feet up as I labored on the toilet. My mother held my leg straight in the air as I lay on my side, a position that I'm quite sure has never made it into any book on pregnancy but was the only position in which I could find any comfort. No less than four people watched as I pooped on the bed while trying to push Naomi out. And let's just say I was less than charitable when the water in the bathtub became uncomfortably cool.

Dan and my mom took turns dropping ice chips into my mouth when I could no longer muster the strength to do it myself. They stood on either side of me and lifted my body when I wanted to change positions. The midwife manually inserted a catheter when I found I was unable to pee on my own. I can still remember the relief and relaxation that swept over my body as someone else emptied my bladder for me. I was as weak and dependent as I've ever been.

At the end of my labor, I lay on the bed a few inches from where I had just pooped with a tiny, wet version of my daughter nestled against my breast. There seemed to be a lot of activity around me, but my brain wasn't registering much, as if it had fallen out with the baby. But I remember my mother appearing at my side with striking clarity. She handed me a glass of orange juice that she had just squeezed herself. She had tears in her eyes.

"You are so strong," she said. "You are so, so strong."

She had just watched me moan, snap, poop, and wander around naked. She had held my legs. I had depended on her. I had let her see my weakness, but she hadn't seen it as such.

"You are so strong," she said.

Until we are willing to step out on faith and let others support us in our weakness, we will never know the miraculous strength of God within us. Second Corinthians 12:9 says, "My grace is sufficient for you, for my power is made perfect in weakness." As we learn to trust the unseen God to meet our needs through the people around us, we learn that our weakness can be the site of our greatest strength. Having faith means letting other people hold up our legs when we can't hold them up for ourselves. The mystery of faith is that depending on someone for that very intimate help is not a sign of weakness, but a sign of a very deep and powerful strength.

11
Waiting Well

—

"Therefore keep watch, because you do not know the day or the hour."

MATTHEW 25:13

I DISTINCTLY REMEMBER MY MOTHER TELLING me that arriving five minutes before an appointment means you are "on time." Planning to arrive "on time" means you will probably be late. A lifetime of this teaching combines with my type-A personality to yield a dizzy sweat when I, my husband, someone I'm meeting with, or anyone I feel vaguely responsible for is late.

I assumed that after decades of arriving on time, my body would have picked up on my habits and would deliver my child a few days prior to my due date. My mother gave birth to me two weeks early, and I had been told that my mother's labor patterns were one indication of what mine might be. I started having intense contractions two weeks before my due date. After a week of those, my mom drove from her home in Tennessee to ours in North Carolina. She had planned to stay with us for one month after the baby was born. Arriving a few days early couldn't hurt.

I had been teaching, but the semester had ended. I had washed and folded the baby's clothes. Her crib was assembled. The diapers were folded, awaiting use. When Mom arrived there was little left to do. We counted our blessings and headed to the pool for some much needed relaxation. The next day was much the same. Everything still seemed ready. By the third day Mom was getting restless, so we made a trip to Target to buy one more type of diaper cream just in case the baby disliked the type we already had. By the afternoon, I was back at the pool and Mom was deep-cleaning our freezer.

Four days later, our house was cleaner than it had ever been, and Mom and I were back at the pool. The lifeguard was typical—a college-age guy with sandy-blond hair and impeccably toned muscles. He had been eyeing us with suspicion for the last week. That afternoon, he stared unabashedly as I waddled onto the glaring concrete. I had been given a bright red maternity bathing suit that had actually looked quite chic two months prior. But that day my bathing suit had given up the fight, and the bottom few inches of my veiny, engorged stomach peeped out at the noonday sun. The lifeguard approached and I reached for my ID, grumbling to myself that I was sure he had noticed our presence every day of the previous week. But instead of asking for ID, he smiled.

"Are you pregnant?" he asked. The innocent expression on his sunny face betrayed a lack of knowledge about all things pregnancy related. I nodded my assent, astonished that even a college guy still needed to ask.

"When are you due?" he continued.

I knew my answer was not the one he hoped to hear. I mustered my most assuring smile and replied, "Today."

He looked as if his life were in immediate danger. His eyes filled with fear. He backed away one bare foot at a time. He suggested that maybe we should be at the hospital instead of the pool, and I quickly tried to explain that babies don't really come on their due dates. My explanation was doing nothing to assuage his growing discomfort, so we finally told him that he would not be responsible for any baby-related activity that might begin at the pool.

Babies don't come on time. Somewhere in the back of my mind, I had a vague idea that a child couldn't be expected to arrive on exactly the date given. But I was completely unprepared for the horrifying news that a baby can safely arrive anywhere between thirty-seven and forty-two weeks gestation. "You can expect your baby anywhere between early May and mid-June," my midwife had cheerily explained. My heart sank. I knew I did not have that type of patience.

"Keep watch, because you do not know the day or the hour," says Jesus.

In Matthew's Gospel, Jesus tells a story about waiting for the kingdom of God. There are ten virgins waiting to greet their bridegroom. They wait and wait, but he doesn't come. Night comes, and they all fall asleep. At midnight a cry rings out, "The bridegroom is here!" The ten virgins all wake up, but it turns out only five of them came prepared. Five brought oil for their lamps, and five had to run to the store to get more oil. The five who run to the store miss the wedding banquet. Jesus ends his story saying, "Keep watch, because you do not know the day or the hour" (Matt. 25:1–13).

The story is a warning to all of Jesus' followers. We must be prepared for Jesus to come. A passive, falling-asleep, unprepared waiting is not enough. There is work to be done! We must create hospitable conditions for Jesus to enter our lives and our world. Jesus chooses a negative example; a story about how *not* to wait. But he could have told a story about how to wait well by simply trading in the virgins for some pregnant women.

Pregnant women surely would have fallen asleep (probably before the virgins) but by the time the bridegroom came, they would have woken up twice to pee and once for a little snack of peanut butter toast and milk. When the bridegroom came striding in at midnight, at least three lamps would already be on. The pregnant woman struggling with insomnia would welcome him to the kitchen table for a midnight cup of herbal tea. The second-time mom would motion the bridegroom to the couch while she finished nursing her firstborn. And the third-time mom would say with a large dose of exasperation, "It's about time you got here—my six-year-old can't sleep for excitement about this wedding feast!" All of them would have their hospital bags packed and waiting by the door. Jesus could have said, "Wait like a pregnant woman."

In all seriousness, pregnancy teaches us exactly the sort of active waiting Jesus asks of us. For nine months or more, we prepare for the coming of a little baby. We change our lives in anticipation of one who will further alter us in ways we cannot imagine. This active waiting begins in the first days. The only sign I had of my child's existence was a pink line on a pee stick, yet I immediately changed my diet. I felt my stomach every morning, waiting for some sign of a growing knot. I waited eagerly from week sixteen to week twenty-one to feel my child kick. But as I waited, even when there were no signs of life, I actively prepared for my child's arrival. I began creating a space in our home where she would feel welcome. I researched what sorts of things would help keep her safe. I planned with my husband for a name that might offer our daughter a vision for who she might become.

My body also practiced this sort of active, prepared waiting. Sciatic nerve pain and an inability to sit anywhere for more than thirty minutes signaled that my ligaments were loosening. My hips were slowly separating to make room for my baby to enter the world. The three weeks of contractions I had prior to my daughter's birth were once called "false labor." I was encouraged by my midwife's use of the term *prelabor* and her explanation that my body was doing what it needed to do to be ready for the baby's arrival.

But active waiting is more than simple preparation. Waiting for my coming daughter meant learning to live with a driving desire for an event that I couldn't control. I desired relief from the pain of pregnancy and the anticipated pain of labor. I desired to meet the little person who had so radically changed my life, and I desired the start of the new life I would have with her. Waiting for a child meant waiting for the fulfillment of a promised blessing I didn't deserve and a coming burden I couldn't imagine. In my final weeks of pregnancy, not knowing when my daughter would come meant that every moment could be the moment she came. This is how Jesus wants us to wait for him.

I wanted each moment to be the start of labor so badly that I thought about it all the time. Such intense, continuous, unfulfilled desire can be paralyzing. I remember sitting in the living room with my mom some eight days after Naomi was due, saying, "All I want to do is go into labor. I can't even begin to think of doing anything else." At the same time, just sitting around was driving me crazy. Thirty minutes later, I found myself yelling, "I have to get out of this house!" I had to learn to let my desire for the start of labor nurture and fuel my preparation instead of immobilizing it. By week forty-two, not knowing the day or the hour had become a lifestyle. I was keeping watch and getting readier by the minute. Before I experienced it, I never knew such waiting was possible. I certainly had never considered waiting for Jesus like that.

The four Gospels each talk about the coming of Christ a little differently. Only two of them actually tell us about Jesus' birth. But all four Gospels paint a vivid picture of John the Baptist as the one who prepares the way for Jesus to come. All four portray John the Baptist as the one who cries out in the wilderness, "Prepare the way for the Lord!" For all of their disagreements, all four Gospels insist that Jesus can't just show up. We need to be prepared. Someone needs to make sure things are ready. John's cry comes from Isaiah 40:3–5. The passage reads:

> A voice of one calling:
> "In the wilderness prepare
> the way for the LORD;
> make straight in the desert
> a highway for our God.
> Every valley shall be raised up,
> every mountain and hill made low;
> the rough ground shall become level,
> the rugged places a plain.

And the glory of the LORD will be revealed,

and all people will see it together."

In its original context, Isaiah is writing to a defeated people who have been taken from their homes by force to live as captives in a foreign land. He is imagining the Lord leading the Israelites back through the desert to their homeland. Isaiah is so firm in his belief that he also imagines how it will be accomplished. If the Lord is going to restore the people to their homes, they'll need a mighty big highway. Isaiah imagines a situation in which the people partner with God for their own deliverance. God will save us, but we have to build the road to enable God's arrival.

Isaiah 40:3–5 is a passage that we read during the liturgical season of Advent, the four weeks leading up to Christmas. Advent is the time when the church waits for the celebration of Jesus' birth—when we set aside time to learn the kind of waiting Jesus asks of us. We read the stories in Luke about Mary's pregnancy. We sing with her the hymn of praise she uses to describe her joy at bearing baby Jesus. We take up Isaiah's cry for an active preparation, a massive construction project that will allow Jesus to enter the world. We get ready together for the coming of a baby who has changed and will change everything about how we live. You might say that it is during Advent that we all act pregnant together. Advent is to the church calendar what weeks thirty-six through forty are to expectant mothers.

I love Advent. I am the first one at the Christmas tree lot the day after Thanksgiving. I have a growing stash of Christmas CDs, some that my mother taught me to love and others I've discovered myself. I have treats that I only cook at Christmas and decorations that only come out to mark this special time of year. We change our home entirely in joyful expectancy of Jesus' birth.

My love for the Christmas season has escalated now that I have children to share in my excitement. This year I found myself wanting to light the third Advent candle in the second week of Advent. I shamefully goaded my two-year-old into asking my husband if we could open just one present early (two weeks before Christmas). I even found myself running through the house squealing, "I can't wait for Santa to come!" Rationally, I know that I will be the one to fill the stockings and place presents under the tree. But even now that I get to be Santa, seeing Santa's magic on Christmas morning still elicits my excited anticipation.

Clearly, I'm not a patient person. I actually have trouble waiting for my toast to pop out of the toaster. Truth be told, I frequently pop it out early and eat it half done, the cold butter perched perkily atop semiwarm bread. Thankfully, I don't think patience is actually a requirement of the kind of waiting Jesus asks of us. At least, not patience as we normally understand it.

We envision patient people as quiet people. They wait in line without complaining even when the cashier has clearly gone on a smoke break without procuring a replacement. Patient people smile sweetly when their children throw tantrums in the grocery store. They lift their children off the floor and explain the consequences of fit throwing in a tone that is gentle but a bit firm and entirely rational. Patient people don't even think about opening Christmas presents two weeks before Christmas. Patient people say with limpid, not-so-understanding smiles, "Patience is a virtue," to those of us who want to open said presents just a touch too early. I don't think anyone has ever called me patient even once in my whole life. Patient people call my husband patient all the time (with the not-so-subtle subtext that he should win an award for putting up with not-so-patient me).

I was taught that patience was at the heart of Christian living from a very young age. I couldn't have been more than six years old when my grandmother taught us a song that goes:

> The fruit of the spirit's not a banana.
> The fruit of the spirit's not a banana.
> The fruit of the spirit's not a banana.

The fruits are love, joy, peace, patience, kindness,
    goodness, faithfulness,
gentleness, and self-contro-o-ol.
Love, joy, peace, patience, kindness, goodness,
    faithfulness, gentleness, and self-control.

Imagine us kids raising our hands above our heads and tilting our bodies in banana-shaped curves during the first three lines. Then imagine us singing verse after verse, inserting every fruit our six-year-old brains could conjure.

The list of spiritual fruits comes from Galatians 5:22–23. My grandfather was a preacher, and one Sunday morning when we were visiting my grandparents, he preached this text. I was delighted to recognize the Scripture, and I sang the words in my head as my grandfather read them from the pulpit. But right after peace, as I was singing "patience," my grandfather read "long-suffering." Long-suffering? That's not how the song goes! I grabbed the King James Bible from the pew in front of me and looked up the verse. Galatians 5:22 began, "But the fruit of the spirit is love, joy, peace, *longsuffering* . . . " I left the Bible open on my lap so I could check it again and again. I was shocked. In my elementary school mind, patience and long-suffering were not the same thing. The quiet people who waited calmly in line at the grocery store were not suffering. The people who blithely waited for Christmas, unphased by the bright packages under the tree, weren't suffering.

If *patience* can be translated "long-suffering," maybe patience isn't what I understood it to be. The truth is, the Bible is much more interested in long-suffering than in any sort of quietism or passive line waiting. The Bible doesn't say much about the attitude we should have while we wait for Jesus. But the Bible is clear that we will endure suffering while we pursue and wait for God's kingdom of justice and love to come fully on earth. Jesus hasn't come quickly, and many of his most faithful children have suffered long and hard. If we want to make it to the metaphorical midnight, maybe we need the fruit of long-suffering more than the attitude we call patience.

Pregnancy's waiting is much more like long-suffering than patience. If the baby is the Christmas present, pregnant women try to rip off that wrapping paper as early as they can. Patience as we know it is nowhere in sight. Trying to "walk out" their babies, women circle neighborhood streets in fiendish haste. I've known women who've gotten acupuncture, massage, and even a special form of chiropractic manipulation to induce labor. At week thirty-eight, women eat spicy food, chocolate cake, and whatever their best friend ate the night before she went into labor. My yoga teacher told me about a magical spot two finger-widths above the inside anklebone that would stimulate labor if massaged firmly. My mother gave me a thumb-size bruise in our ardent application of this tactic.

But no matter how "impatient" pregnant women can be, they know how to suffer long and hard as they actively prepare for the coming of new life into the world. In those last weeks of pregnancy, pain shot through my lower back and thigh every time I stood up. But I still got up to wash Naomi's diapers, and I still stood to hang them on the line in preparation for her first poops and pees. Insomnia kept my brain alert and ticking in the obscenely early-morning hours that I would come to know too well in the coming years. But I still rested at night, fighting off the urges toward midnight cabinet rearranging, because I knew Naomi needed me to be rested for her labor and delivery whenever it came.

Pregnancy teaches just the sort of long-suffering, active waiting that we need for the life of faith. It's not easy to be long-suffering. It's not easy to prepare each day for the arrival of one who refuses to share his estimated time of arrival. It's not easy to turn a driving expectancy into fuel for active preparation. I don't want to wait like that. But pregnancy demands it. The life of faith demands it too. But the life of faith isn't quite so controlling as our pregnant bodies. In pregnancy, we are forced to wait. In the life of faith, we can actually avoid active waiting for Jesus. Most of us do. We choose not to think of his coming at all over the disappointment of longing for him only to have him not appear at the end of the day. We avoid asking questions like:

What kind of baby clothes does Jesus need?

Who needs to be on my e-mail list announcing
his upcoming birth?

What sorts of daily habits will ensure his ability
to live in my life?

How can I make my home a safe and welcoming place
for Jesus, particularly if he arrives in the form
of the stranger, widow, or orphan (as he says
he will)?

We have to choose to practice the active waiting we learn
in pregnancy when it comes to the life of faith.

It was a week before Christmas. My friends Jonathan
and Leah were waiting for Jesus, but they were much more
avidly waiting for Norah Ann, the new little girl growing
inside Leah's tummy. Leah had been struggling with high
blood pressure for about a month. She kept testing negative
for preeclampsia, but the midwives were worried it could
develop at any moment. She was ordered on strict bed rest,
and she had to test her blood pressure each day.

The blood pressure tests seemed to be going better than the
bed rest until she was told that if her blood pressure didn't
go down, she would be induced at the end of the week. That
got Leah quickly into bed. The end of the week came and,
miraculously, Leah's blood pressure was down. She was

sent home to continue her rest and blood pressure checking until Norah came in her own due time. I called Leah a few days before Christmas.

"What are you doing?" I asked.

"Waiting for Norah," she replied.

I laughed and she went on to explain that she was actually waiting for another load of hand-me-down baby clothes to come out of the wash. As we chatted, passing a few of the moments until Norah's birth, Leah explained something of what it felt to have expected Norah's arrival a few days ago and yet still be pregnant.

"This blood pressure scare made me realize that we weren't really prepared. All of a sudden we realized we had clothes to wash and diapers to fold and a bag to pack. But now we feel ready," she explained. I laughed again.

"I don't mean to laugh," I said, "I just don't think you can ever really be *ready* for a baby."

"Well, I say 'ready,' but then we find six more things to do the next day."

Perhaps this is just what Jesus asks. I don't think we can ever really be "ready" for Jesus' coming. But we can practice the active, expectant waiting of pregnant women in our lives of faith. We can create a hospitable space for Jesus to come into our homes. And then we can still find six more things to do for Jesus the next day.

12
A Different Sort of Worship

"And a little child will lead them."
ISAIAH 11:6

I NEVER EXPECTED PREGNANCY TO AFFECT my spiritual life. I was grateful to God for the child growing inside of me. I prayed for the baby's safety and my own. I prayed that God would teach me and Dan to be faithful parents. I assumed pregnancy was a natural and joyful part of life, and I planned to walk with God through it as I had walked through other joyous experiences in the past.

But shortly into my first pregnancy, my spiritual life stopped working. There was no drastic shift, no crisis of faith, no problems with the baby. I simply found myself with no energy. While I was able to accept my new limitations in most aspects of my life, I felt confused and guilty that this lack of energy extended to my relationship with God. I assumed my friends would understand that my new eight o'clock bedtime would preclude our previous levels of communication, but I wondered about telling God I was too tired to talk. I felt no guilt about skimming through my reading for work or bowing out of volunteer activities, but could I really back down on Bible reading or skip my community's daily prayer times?

I hoped that as I settled into pregnancy I would settle into a pregnant walk with God. To my dismay, no settling occurred. The less energy I had in general, the less energy I had for my traditional spiritual disciplines. By the third trimester, being awake for morning or evening prayer was almost laughable. My personal Bible reading was infrequent at best. When Lent rolled around, I could not imagine adding another ascetic practice to the laundry list of foods and drinks I was already avoiding for the baby's health. I still prayed each night, but I was disappointed at how personal and needy my prayers had become. I felt like a spiritual weakling praying for relief from my nausea when I was quite sure there were global concerns of peace and justice that my prayers could have been addressing. Try as I might, I couldn't stay awake long enough to pry my prayers off my own pains or the safety of the little one growing inside me.

To make matters worse, Sunday morning worship seemed almost intentional in its hostility to my new pregnant self. How could I be expected to sit and stand for one to three hours with nothing to eat or drink and no place to prop my feet? Was I really supposed to invest in a whole new wardrobe of Sunday dresses? Why did we have to dress up to come to worship anyway? I found these and a host of other questions crowding out any thoughts of God as I sat in the pew each week.

One Sunday, after a sermon on the importance of taking time for God each day no matter what you have going on or how tired you are at night, we were instructed to rise for the hymn of invitation. I rose dutifully, thinking about how the preacher had obviously never been pregnant, and as I opened my mouth to sing the first note, black spots blurred my vision. A wave of dizziness washed over me, and my lungs seemed unable to expand enough to take in air. I sunk back into the pew, looked down at my swollen feet, and thought to myself, "I quit."

I made my way out of the sanctuary and lay on the floor of the church library. I left the lights off and lay between the tables, hoping that no one would see me. Waves of anger and guilt and exhaustion crashed into one another and salty tears dampened my face. Why couldn't I get it together? Why should I have to get it together? What had happened to all of my spiritual practices? Was I just lazy? Was Christianity inherently unfriendly to pregnant women? Where was God in all of this fatigue? How could I be losing my relationship with God when I most wanted to be celebrating with God over this great gift I was being given?

My husband found me pathetically slumped between the tables. He lifted me up and promised that we would find a way to make church work for me. I leaned against him, grateful that someone else was going to help me carry the burden of my spiritual life, and we went home for a nap.

That day began a number of Sunday morning experiments. We started small, agreeing to drive to church instead of walking. Then we decided to sit down for the hymns and bring a bottle of water into the sanctuary. Then Dan started making me a small snack for before and after worship. I had been conflicted about attending a prenatal yoga class that met during the Sunday school hour, but Dan encouraged me to go. We found that if I brought a change of clothes and he picked me up in the car, we had just enough time to make it to worship. That hour of yoga was the best my body felt all week, and it drastically improved my mood at church. We even experimented with "dressing down" for worship. I wore comfortable shoes and mustered the courage to simply add a nice shirt to my yoga pants on a few blessed Sundays. Dan helped by dressing down himself.

I was slowly learning to accept God's grace through my husband. I was beginning to live into a kinder, gentler, less rigorous practice of my faith. And yet, as the heat of our North Carolina summer converged with my ninth month, I still struggled on Sunday mornings. One such morning I was lying on the bed in my underwear. I was lying on my side because lying on my back delivered the sensation of a boulder crushing my lungs. But even with the pillow-assisted positioning and a fan blowing directly on me, I couldn't seem to create conditions amenable to breathing.

"Dan," I moaned, stretching his name into a whiny three syllables, "I cannot put on any clothes. I cannot stand up. I cannot breathe. I cannot go to church."

I looked up, desperately hoping that he would have the magical suggestion for how to make this "okay." He stood still, quietly pondering the situation, and just when I was sure he was about to heroically rally me out of bed and into my least constricting sundress, he took off his shirt.

"Great!" he exclaimed. "Let's just lie here and read the Bible." He exuded confidence in this decision, and I let his assurance push aside my worry about whether or not lying on the bed naked constituted legitimate worship. After we read the lectionary passages for the day, we lay side by side.

"This is just like Adam and Eve," he said with a smile.

I smiled back with a big, incredulous, grateful smile. I wondered at the woman I was becoming. I wondered at this new sort of worship. And I wondered at the husband and new baby that were teaching me to worship in this new way. It was our first Adam and Eve Sunday, and it was good, very good indeed.

By my second pregnancy, I was becoming more comfortable with my relaxed faith. I was more willing to listen to my body and to my baby, and I believed that God would find ways to continue our relationship with my new limitations. So one Sunday, when we were on a retreat with our community and it was clear that my daughter Naomi needed a nap right as we were all preparing to leave for church, I volunteered to stay home while she slept.

I sat outside. I read a little from the Bible. Mostly I watched the light bouncing off the water onto the underbellies of the leaves above me. Without thinking, I began to sing, "My soul proclaims thy greatness, oh my God. My spirit rejoices in God my savior." As I began to repeat the song, Fay began to dance inside of me, and I mean really dance. These were not little kicks. She was full on rolling and tumbling. I was singing. She was dancing. We were worshiping together. So I began to sing, "*Our* souls proclaim your greatness, oh our God. Our spirits rejoice in God our savior." Fay continued to dance. When I finally fell silent, she fell still. I prayed a prayer of thanksgiving, thanking God for giving me the gift of worshiping with this little daughter that I hadn't even seen yet. Only later did I realize that the song God had placed on my heart was the same song that Mary sang when she was pregnant with Jesus.

Luke tells the story of how Mary goes to visit her relative Elizabeth after an angel tells her they are both with child. Luke writes:

At that time Mary got ready and hurried to a town in the hill country of Judea, where she entered Zechariah's home and greeted Elizabeth. When Elizabeth heard Mary's greeting, the baby leaped in her womb, and Elizabeth was filled with the Holy Spirit. In a loud voice she exclaimed, "Blessed are you among women, and blessed is the child you will bear! But why am I so favored, that the mother of my Lord should come to me? As soon as the sound of your greeting reached my ears, the baby in my womb leaped for joy. Blessed is she who has believed that the Lord would fulfill his promises to her!" (Lk. 1:39–45)

I love this story. It overflows with joy: joy over pregnancy and joy over the Lord Jesus coming into the world. When I read of baby John the Baptist leaping around in Elizabeth's tummy, I remember what it was like to have Fay dance in my own womb. Luke makes a radical claim here. He seems to suggest that baby John is able to recognize Mary and baby Jesus. Luke suggests that this little fetal John knows the truth about Jesus and leaps about it. Not only does John recognize Jesus, but he teaches his mother the truth about who Jesus is. Because of John's leaping, Elizabeth is the first person in Luke's Gospel to proclaim the lordship of Christ. John's leaping fills Elizabeth with the Holy Spirit and she becomes the first person to preach the good news that Jesus is Lord of all the earth.

Elizabeth's shouts of joy prompt Mary to sing. Mary sings a song that Christians have come to call the Magnificat. It begins with the line that I sang with Fay. She sings a song of praise for all the great things God has done, but her song also highlights that God will take care of those who are in need. She sings of God as one who loves the humble, feeds the hungry, and remembers to help God's servants. Mary's song highlights the kinds of things we learn about God in pregnancy.

In pregnancy, I quickly learned that my relationship with God was not dependent on my own strength or my own ability to perform religious rituals. I was humbled (and embarrassed) about my own limits, but in that humbling I experienced God sustaining our relationship in spite of my limitations. I learned the truth that my salvation, even my worship, is given to me as a gift. I cannot force it to happen. I cannot compel myself to have the energy for it, any more than I could compel Fay to worship with me that day. But I can receive the gift of time with God when it comes. And I can sing joyfully of God's goodness when I do get to experience those moments.

To learn a new way of worshiping in our pregnancies we have to believe that our unborn babies can be our teachers. Fay and Naomi have indeed taught me my own hunger, weakness, humility, and need for help. Those are lessons that I can imagine a baby teaching from the womb. But Luke claims that our babies might also be able to recognize Jesus and prompt us to tell truths about Jesus that we might not have known otherwise. Even after my experience of worshiping with Fay, I still have trouble imagining our babies as that sort of teacher. We simply do not have models in our culture for learning about Jesus the way Elizabeth does from baby John.

Isaiah proclaims that when God's kingdom comes on earth, "a little child will lead [us]" into it (11:6). If we can bring ourselves to believe that, we can learn a whole new way of being with God during our pregnancies. But in reality, it is very difficult to let our children teach us how to worship. It was hard for me to listen to the demands of my babies over the demands of Christian tradition. It was hard for me to learn from my weakness when it seemed to mean giving up on my spiritual disciplines. It is still hard for me to worship with my children, especially when it means skipping official worship services. I worry that I'm being a bad Christian. I worry that I'm interpreting the leaps and dancing of my babies wrong. I worry about worrying. But I have heard God respond to my worry over and over again, saying, "Peace. Be still. You are enough."

The most astonishing thing I have learned about worship and discipleship during pregnancy is that I am already doing it. It is okay that I don't have energy for my spiritual practices like daily Bible reading and prayers because spiritual discipline is built into pregnant life. For example, I mentioned being frustrated during Lent of my first pregnancy. I had already given up so much I loved: coffee, soda, junk food, regular use of over-the-counter drugs. I couldn't begin to imagine giving up anything else.

So I didn't.

I have come to believe that my frustrated refusal to add another ascetic practice to my life during Lent was the right choice and could have been made in peace, without guilt or frustration. Sacrifices made during Lent can teach us about our human frailty, our longings and desires, our need for God's help in keeping those commitments. The sacrifices of pregnancy can teach us the same things (except for the duration of nine months instead of one!). The practices of pregnancy are the practices of Lent. Nothing needs to be added.

While my intentional prayer time dwindled during pregnancy, I came closer to "praying without ceasing" than ever before or since. I would find myself praying without even intending to—for the health and safety of the child growing within me, for her future, for her safe delivery, for my role as her mother. I sunk into Sabbath rest with necessity and relief. I delighted in the details of the child God was creating within me. I learned to wait for the birth of a child like no Advent or Christmas had ever been able to teach. I began to understand the mystery at the heart of our faith: that suffering for the sake of another can indeed bring forth new life.

I learned all of this without any intentional, religious effort. My baby taught me these faith lessons by simply living within me. The good news of walking with God while you are with child is that you are already doing it. You do not have to conjure up energy that you do not have. What you are doing is enough.

As with any spiritual disciplines, there are ways to deepen your practice. There are ways to add intentionality to what you are doing. There are even ways to challenge yourself if you have the energy and desire to do so. Most of the ways I felt called to challenge myself and add to what I was already doing were through prayer. For one month of my pregnancy with Naomi, I felt convicted that every time I prayed for Naomi's health and safety, I should add a prayer for the health and safety of other children. Sometimes I prayed for children in our neighborhood, sometimes for children around the world. It took no more than twenty seconds each time, but it was a way for me to expand my prayer life beyond myself and my baby. During the last month of my pregnancy with Fay, I found myself ardently wishing at least once an hour that she would come. We had entered Advent, and I felt convicted about how much I desired her arrival and how little I thought about Jesus' upcoming birth. I committed to pray the short historic Christian prayer, "Come, Lord Jesus," every time I found myself exclaiming, "Come on, Fay!"

These little commitments to prayer were important to me, but they were not necessary. The ideas to do them came as a gift, and the energy to pray the additional prayers came as a gift as well. Receiving my faith as a gift is still difficult for me. I feel like I should be doing something. I want faith to feel like an accomplishment. I expect my worship to be hard work. I have trouble letting my daily care for my children be worship enough. I have trouble giving in to Dan's appeals for another Adam and Eve Sunday.

But as I've moved from the exhaustion of pregnancy to the exhaustion of parenting toddlers, I've found daily reason to consider accepting God's gracious offer that worship might be found in what I'm already doing. Even though I wrestle my girls into dresses and bows on most Sundays, I've learned to accept that Adam and Eve Sunday is sometimes enough. I am slowly learning that it is more than enough. It is, as God proclaimed about the first Sunday, very good indeed.

One Last Thing . . .

IF YOU'VE MADE IT THIS FAR, you've probably noticed that I love the Bible. But if you've made it this far, you've probably also noticed that I get cranky quite easily. And I'll be honest, there are parts of the Bible that have historically made me so cranky that it takes every little shard of my self-constraint not to rip pages right out of my worn-out, leather-bound NIV.

Page 1258 is one of the pages I've wanted to rip out. In my Bible, that page is the home of 1 Timothy 2. In it, the author explains that women should be quiet, not teach, take off their jewelry, submit to men, and, for the love of God, not do anything so flagrantly sinful as braid their hair. The chapter ends with the phrase, "But women will be saved through child-bearing—if they continue in faith, love and holiness with propriety."

As a woman pastor, this is one of those chapters that gets flung in my face with some frequency. I have heard this passage used to justify why women shouldn't work outside the home, why women should have as many babies as they physically can, why women are less spiritually capable than men, and why mothering should be at the tip top of every woman's list of concerns. Lovers of this passage are eager to say not only that childbearing is one way that women might know God, but that childbearing is the *only*, or at least the *predominant*, way that women can know God.

I have spent this book describing some of the ways that women come to know God in childbearing. I have gone a step further to name women as God's partners in the work of pregnancy and labor. I have tried to show how women become the very image of Christ as they welcome others into their bodies, give their blood as food, and suffer for the sake of new life. I have claimed that pregnancy might teach us the very disciplines we need to live the life of faith. In short, I've argued myself into the truth hiding behind 1 Timothy 2:15.

If salvation is about being made into the image of God, then women can be saved through childbearing. If salvation means learning to let Jesus live in you with all the hungry and naked little ones he brings along, then women are saved in childbearing. If being saved means coming to know God's love for you as you learn to extend that love to others, then women are drenched with salvation in childbearing.

Like it or not, I have to name the way that 1 Timothy is right. I want to name how wildly important and holy the work of pregnancy is, but in naming its importance, I don't want to say it is the only or most important work women can do. I came to know God well before my reproductive organs were fully functioning. I was ordained as a Baptist minister before I was married. I stood at the Lord's Table, in the place of Christ, and offered the body and blood of Jesus to a congregation before I ever offered my bones and blood to Naomi and Fay as food. I have been given a profound way of knowing God in my pregnancies, but I've been given that same gift in myriad other ways.

Some women can't have children. Some women choose not to. Some women nurture new life through adoption. And I understand that all of those women will be given the gift of partnering with God time and time again in different, beautiful, life-giving ways. We worship a God of endless possibility.

For me, the mind-blowing good news of this book is not that pregnancy is the only way to get to know God, but that pregnancy is way of knowing God at all. I count it no small miracle that God meets us in our constipation, groaning, and back pain and says our suffering mirrors God's own. I am delighted that God meets us in our neurotic planning, pregnancy book reading, and ultrasound gazing and says that we are learning to love the way God loves us. I adore the God who meets us as we change our daily habits, believe fiercely in an unseen little master, and impatiently count off the days until delivery and says those are just the habits we need to live the life of faith. We do indeed worship a God of endless possibility.

I hope you go from this book encouraged. I hope that you can look in the mirror and know that the more bloated you get, the more you glow with the light of the Transfiguration. I hope you are empowered to know that you are taking up God's creative work. I hope that empowerment makes sciatic nerve pain easier to bear. I hope you can see the image of God in the women around you. I even dare to hope that you'll be able to glimpse the image of God in yourself. I hope these things for you. I hope them for myself. I hope them for every woman who labors to bring new life to the world.

I hope you go forth in peace. May the love of a mothering God, the peace of a nursing Christ, and the fellowship of a groaning Spirit go with you. Amen.

Acknowledgments

If it takes a village to raise children, it takes all of the villagers' extended friends and family for a mother raising children to write a book. I have a lot of people to thank.

First, to everyone who gave me space to write by caring for Naomi and Fay. Vern, Leah, Beth, Tomi, Anne Marie, and Matt, I'm glad my daughters get to spend time with you. You are a gift to our family, and this book could not have been written without the time you gave me. And to Dan, while its part of your job description to take care of our children, thank you for donating your breaks to the cause. I remain as thankful as ever for a life-partner who understands our vocation communally.

There are a number of people who read this book in its various forms. And I want to say thank you to each of you in turn . . .

To my editor, Jon, and all those who helped me at Paraclete Press. You took a chance on a first-time author, braved my deluge of e-mails, and responded graciously and helpfully. Thank you for making this project a reality.

To Lisa, Holly, Jasmine, Jenny, Becca, Leah, Amy Laura, Dan, and Matt. Thank you for being my e-mail support group. Your assurances that you laughed, cried, and heard my voice while reading were the best feedback I could have ever gotten. Your encouragement kept me writing. It astounds me that your support in this project is only a fraction of the support you've each offered me throughout my life. Thank you.

To Jonathan, who made writing look so easy that I could imagine myself doing it. Of course, it wasn't as easy as you made it look, so thank you for stepping in and helping me when I realized the difficulty of the work that flows so gorgeously and prolifically out of you.

To Lauren, my book doula, who was available by text every hour that I labored to give birth to this book. You offered me more help than I would have ever felt comfortable asking of you. You even had the grace to pass your wisdom along with a large dose of friendship. God looked down and saw my need for sarcastic conversation at a cozy window table and sent you.

To my mom, who was my first example of how much mothers can look like God. You're still the clearest reflection of Christ that I have ever seen. You taught me to write. You read my drafts. You're in half the stories in this book. I owe this book (and life as I know it) to you. I hope you can forgive my use of the word *turd*.

And to the God who came to earth and took a chance on looking like us. In so doing, you gave us the chance to look like you. It seems like a crazy way of going about things, but seeing visions of you in the women and men around me has filled my life with unspeakable beauty. I hope you can hear my gratitude in the words of this book. Thank you.

Notes

Chapter 1: Co-Creating with God

3. *"I have created a man with God!"* This is my own translation of Genesis 4:1. Unless otherwise noted, all biblical quotations in this book are taken from the New International Version of the Bible.

8. *Eve uses the word* create *to describe her work.* The verb used here comes from the Hebrew root word *qanah*. It can be translated "to acquire," hence the standard biblical translations. But whenever *qanah* is used in the Bible to refer to God's actions, we translate it as "create." When the Bible calls God "Creator," it most often comes from this root word. When we read in Psalm 139:13, "For you created my inmost being; you knit me together in my mother's womb," the word for "create" comes from *qanah*. When used of God, this verb is most often translated "create," not "acquire." I am suggesting that Eve, or the author of her narrative, is choosing language suggestively. *Qanah* is a word that on one level means "acquire." On another level, it is a word that is associated with God's creative activity.

We can translate in a way that acknowledges Eve as a co-creator with God, or we can translate in a way that makes Eve seem more a recipient of the child she grew and bore. I choose to translate in line with the former.

Chapter 3: Learning to Rest

41. *"It is a day on which we are called upon*   Abraham Joshua Heschel, *Sabbath* (New York: Farrar, Straus, and Giroux, 1951), 10.

Chapter 6: Suffering and New Life

78. *Amnesty International produced a report*   A full text and summary of the report "Deadly Delivery: The Maternal Health Care Crisis in the USA" is available for free at www.amnestyusa.org.

85. *Curse becomes the blessing of new life,*   I want to take a moment to acknowledge the danger of seeing Christ in women's experiences of suffering. By danger, I mean the actual physical danger that women have faced when religious authorities have encouraged them to accept various forms of suffering as Christ accepted the cross. I am most troubled, specifically, by how this logic is used in situations of domestic violence. In my work as a pastor I have met too many women who stayed in abusive relationships because they were

encouraged to accept their suffering as Christ accepted his. Such encouragement can be a death sentence. I want to be clear that I think the best way for women in abusive relationships to image Christ is by escaping their persecutors in the same way that Jesus eluded angry mobs when it wasn't his time to suffer.

Everything we suffer will not be the cross. Some of it will just be injustice. For our suffering to be like Christ's, it must bring new life to the world. Seeing an image of Jesus in our own suffering should encourage us. If we are not encouraged or given new life, we should rethink the analogy.

Finally, I want to say clearly that women don't have to die to reflect the suffering of Christ. Most of the time that Paul speaks of taking up the cross in the Bible, he is not referencing physical death. In Romans 12, Paul offers us the powerful idea of becoming "living sacrifices" and encourages us to be transformed into the very body of Christ while we are still living. Pregnant women beautifully embody Paul's idea of a living sacrifice. Death need not be added—the image is already complete.

Chapter 7: Communion and Calcium Deficiency

91. *"My body is real food."*   I use *The New International Reader's Version* here because its language more closely mirrors the Eucharistic liturgy than the *NIV*.

96. *They thought that breast milk was*   Caroline Walker Bynum, *Jesus as Mother: Studies in the Spirituality of the High Middle Ages* (Berkeley: University of California Press, 1982), 132. I highly recommend this book to anyone who finds this imagery of Jesus as mother intriguing and wants to learn more about this metaphor in the history of the church.

97. *Little ones . . . run and throw themselves*   Ibid., 152.

Chapter 8: Expanding Bellies and the Mystery of the Church

108. *There is no other organ quite like*   Ina May Gaskin, *Ina May's Guide to Childbirth* (New York: Random House, 2003), 144.

109. *"O Christ, you have given birth*   Eugene F. Rogers, *After the Spirit: A Constructive Pneumatology from Resources Outside the Modern West* (Grand Rapids, MI: Wm. B. Eerdmans Publishing Co., 2005), 119.

About Paraclete Press

Who We Are

Paraclete Press is a publisher of books, recordings, and DVDs on Christian spirituality. Our publishing represents a full expression of Christian belief and practice—from Catholic to Evangelical, from Protestant to Orthodox.

We are the publishing arm of the Community of Jesus, an ecumenical monastic community in the Benedictine tradition. As such, we are uniquely positioned in the marketplace without connection to a large corporation and with informal relationships to many branches and denominations of faith.

What We Are Doing

Books

Paraclete publishes books that show the richness and depth of what it means to be Christian. Although Benedictine spirituality is at the heart of all that we do, we publish books that reflect the Christian experience across many cultures, time periods, and houses of worship. We publish books that nourish the vibrant life of the church and its people— books about spiritual practice, formation, history, ideas, and customs.

We have several different series, including the best-selling Living Library, Paraclete Essentials, and Paraclete Giants series of classic texts in contemporary English; A Voice from the Monastery—men and women monastics writing about living a spiritual life today; award-winning literary faith fiction and poetry; and the Active Prayer Series that brings creativity and liveliness to any life of prayer.

Recordings

From Gregorian chant to contemporary American choral works, our music recordings celebrate sacred choral music through the centuries. Paraclete distributes the recordings of the internationally acclaimed choir Gloriæ Dei Cantores, praised for their "rapt and fathomless spiritual intensity" by *American Record Guide,* and the Gloriæ Dei Cantores Schola, which specializes in the study and performance of Gregorian chant. Paraclete is also the exclusive North American distributor of the recordings of the Monastic Choir of St. Peter's Abbey in Solesmes, France, long considered to be a leading authority on Gregorian chant.

DVDs

Our DVDs offer spiritual help, healing, and biblical guidance for life issues: grief and loss, marriage, forgiveness, anger management, facing death, and spiritual formation.

Learn more about us at our Web site:
www.paracletepress.com,
or call us toll-free at 1-800-451-5006.

Also available from Paraclete Press

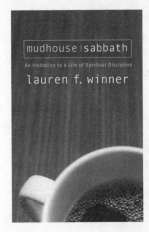

Mudhouse Sabbath

An Invitation to a Life of Spiritual Discipline

by Lauren Winner

ISBN: 978-1-55725-532-7 $14.95, Paperback

Lauren invites Christians to enrich their faith with eleven Jewish spiritual practices from Judaism. Whether discussing attentive eating, candle-lighting, or the differences between the Jewish Sabbath and a Sunday spent at the *Mudhouse*, her favorite coffee shop, Winner writes with appealing honesty and rare insight.

Mudhouse Sabbath DVD

with Lauren Winner

ISBN: 978-1-55725-683-6 $49.99

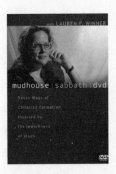

Divided into seven sections or lessons, with discussion topics filmed on location, this 65-minute DVD resource will help you or your study group explore how our faith is rooted in ancient, Jewish, spiritual traditions and ritual. *Mudhouse Sabbath DVD* will challenge you to practice your faith in ways that are biblical, Christ-like, and imminently practical.

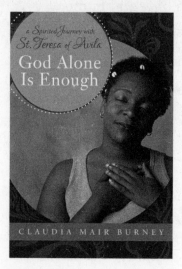

God Alone Is Enough
A Spirited Journey with St. Teresa of Avila

by Claudia Mair Burney

ISBN: 978-1-55725-661-4, $16.99, Paperback

This lively book introduces 21st-century Christians to one of our most endearing prayer warriors, guiding them through her most radical teachings. Here, Teresa of Avila is not a lofty, inaccessible saint; she's a companion, taking readers on a rollicking journey through their own interior castles. The secrets of Teresa's intimate devotional life are revealed, and readers learn practical ways to understand what it means to come to know God and "enjoy" God.

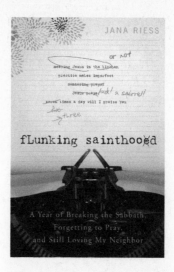

Flunking Sainthood

*A Year of Breaking the Sabbath, Forgetting to Pray,
and Still Loving My Neighbor*

by Jana Riess

ISBN: 978-1-55725-660-7 $16.99, Paperback

*Can an ordinary twenty-first century American become a saint?
No, apparently not. But the most valuable spiritual lessons
often come in our least saintly moments.*

This wry memoir tackles twelve different spiritual practices
in a quest to become more saintly. What emerges is a funny
yet vulnerable story of the quest for spiritual perfection and
the reality of spiritual failure which turns out to be a valuable
practice in and of itself.

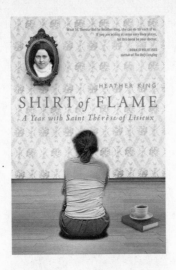

Shirt of Flame

A Year with St. Thérèse of Lisieux

by Heather King

ISBN: 978-1-55725-808-3 $16.99, French Flap

If you have not read Heather King before, her honesty may shock you. In this remarkable memoir, you will see how a convert with a checkered past spends a year reflecting upon St. Thérèse of Lisieux and discovers the radical faith, true love, and abundant life of a cloistered nineteenth-century French nun.

Available from most booksellers or through Paraclete Press:
www.paracletepress.com; 1-800-451-5006.
Try your local bookstore first.